CW00330582

PERSON-CENTRED PRACTICE

case studies in positive psychology

Edited by

Richard Worsley and Stephen Joseph

PCCS BOOKS
Ross-on-Wye

First published in 2007

PCCS Books Ltd
2 Cropper Row
Alton Road
Ross-on-Wye
Herefordshire
HR9 5LA
UK
Tel +44 (0)1989 763 900
www.pccs-books.co.uk

This collection: © Richard Worsley and Stephen Joseph 2007

Chapter 1 © R Worsley and S Joseph, 2007; Chapter 2 © A Payne, 2007;
Chapter 3 © M Campling, 2007; Chapter 4 © G Proctor and A Regan, 2007;
Chapter 5 © T Sanders and J O'Brien, 2007; Chapter 6 © E Catterall, 2007;
Chapter 7 © JD Bozarth and A Glauser, 2007; Chapter 8 © J Hawkins, 2007;
Chapter 9 © R Worsley, 2007; Chapter 10 © M v Kalmthout, 2007;
Chapter 11 © B Krietemeyer and G Prouty, 2007;
Chapter 12 © D Van Werde, 2007;
Chapter 13 © MS Warner, 2007; Chapter 14 © BE Levitt, 2007;
Chapter 15 © G Prouty, 2007; Chapter 16 © P Sanders, 2007;
Chapter 17 © TG Patterson and S Joseph, 2007;
Chapter 18 © S Joseph and R Worsley, 2007.

All rights reserved.
No part of this publication may be reproduced, stored in a retrieval system, transmitted or
utilised in any form by any means, electronic, mechanical, photocopying or recording or
otherwise without permission in writing from the publishers.
The authors have asserted their rights to be identified as the authors of this work in
accordance with the Copyright, Designs and Patents Act 1988.

Person-Centred Practice: Case studies in positive psychology

A CIP catalogue record for this book is available from the British Library

ISBN 978 1 898059 95 0

Cover design by Old Dog Graphics
Printed by Cromwell Press, Trowbridge, UK

DEDICATION

For Tony Merry (1948–2004).
Reader in Psychology, University of East London.
Visionary proponent and scholar of person-centred therapy and editor of the
journal *Person-Centred Practice* (1993–2004). He enabled many practitioners and
scholars to have a first voice in print and in his working with us
there was a gentle wisdom, openness and generosity.

ACKNOWLEDGEMENTS

We would again like to thank Pete Sanders for his faith in our work and for his
suggestions and support along the way; also Helen Dean for her editorial work, both
detailed and humane. Our thanks go to our respective colleagues at the University of
Warwick, the University of Nottingham and City College, Coventry. We have much
appreciated the commitment of our fellow authors of this book. However, our main
debt, in all that we think and have learned, is to our students, clients and supervisees.

CONTENTS

PREFACE

STEPHEN JOSEPH AND RICHARD WORSLEY

Person-centred theory is a meta-theoretical perspective to understanding the human condition. It is a radical and revolutionary perspective that is founded on the assumption that human beings have an inherent tendency towards growth, development and optimal functioning. But these do not happen automatically. For people to actualise their inherent optimal nature they require the right social environment. Without the right social environment the inherent tendency towards growth can become thwarted and usurped, leading instead to psychological distress and dysfunction. The assumption that human beings have an inherent tendency towards growth, development and optimal functioning serves as the guiding principle for client-centred therapeutic practice, even when working with people who are deeply distressed.

Person-centred theory is often misunderstood as superficial and naïve. But nothing could be further from the truth. It is a theory with real depth, which is able to confront the dark side of the human condition as well as the positive aspects. Person-centred theory therefore promises to provide the foundation stone for a new positive psychology of mental health.

In 2005, the publication of our book, *Person-Centred Psychopathology*, put forward the case for a positive psychology of mental health. It included some twenty- three chapters by leading theorists and practitioners from North America, the United Kingdom and Europe. The book covered issues of theory, practice and research. This volume, *Person-Centred Practice*, is a book which can be read wholly in its own right, but which also complements the previous volume. Therapy is above all a practised art. In this volume, senior practitioners and theorists offer case studies through which the insights of the first volume are illustrated, explained and elaborated. We believe that this application of theory into practice is equally important for practitioners, academics and those who are training as therapists, as well as those who need to assess the effectiveness and rationale of person-centred therapy.

Stephen is a psychologist who embraces person-centred theory for grounding his practice and research, and building his theoretical perspectives. He believes that person-centred personality theory offers us the best psychological perspective we have yet of the human condition and a preferable alternative paradigm to the medical model for understanding human distress. Person-centred theory raises questions about our fundamental assumptions about human nature and about the values we hold as professional psychologists, counsellors, and psychotherapists. His purpose over the last few years has been to help begin to bring the ideas of the person-centred approach back into mainstream psychological practice.

Richard's background is as a practitioner and a trainer. He has long been struck by the fact that even beginning counsellors have to make sense of the experiences of a wide range of clients, some of whom present with challenging issues. Both for trainee counsellors and for mature practitioners, the question hovers at the back of the mind: Is my approach adequate to the task? In multidisciplinary settings, the person-centred approach can get a bad press in this respect. Richard has become keen to advocate the approach as a competent and humane way of being. He has learned much from his clients, but above all that the human spirit, rooted in the organism which is our embodied selves, has vast reserves with which to cope creatively in the face of seemingly overwhelming distress. He has particular theoretical interests in process work, in integrative, person-centred practice, and in the philosophy and spirituality of counselling.

This book stands for both of us as a learning about, and an assertion of, the human capacity to grow in the face of adversity. We hope that practitioners, trainers, and those in training in the varied mental health professions will also find the learning and the wisdom in this book of value to them.

CHAPTER 1

CASE STUDIES AND POSITIVE PSYCHOLOGY

RICHARD WORSLEY AND STEPHEN JOSEPH

> Whilst critical psychologists and psychiatrists have been developing their arguments in favour of dismantling the medical model, psychopathology and psychodiagnosis, client-centred therapists have been treading water. As the professionalisation of psychological therapies gathered pace, practitioners were required to be inducted into the lower echelons of the medical model as diagnosticians. Diagnosis became, as John Shlien put it, 'their security blanket as well as their entering wedge'.
>
> (Sanders, 2005: 37)

In *Person-Centred Psychopathology: A positive psychology of mental health* (Joseph and Worsley, 2005), a group of some twenty, internationally-renowned scholars set about demonstrating that the person-centred approach has a deep, subtle and developing theoretical response to client groups who are challenging, and who are often classified by mental health professionals as having one or another psychopathology as described by the Diagnostic and Statistical Manual of the American Psychiatric Association (*DSM-IV-TR:* American Psychiatric Association, 2000), for example.[1] Too often the person-centred approach is stereotyped as lightweight and suitable only for work with the worried well. Nothing, of course, could be further from the truth. It is merely that the approach is widely misunderstood—sometimes innocently, occasionally wilfully—perhaps because it is effective and radical, and challenges the presuppositions of the medical model.

The medical model is embedded in some parts of the world of counselling and psychotherapy, but even more so in the statutory sector of the mental health industry. It is protected in this privilege by those with a vested interest: those who fund mental health practice and who take refuge in the pseudo-science of objective and impersonal symptomatology; the pharmaceutical industry whose profits depend in part on the treatment of human distress as if it were a disease; and even those of us from within the person-centred approach, who, as Shlien's words at the head of this chapter make clear, take refuge in a pseudo-professionalism which adopts, uncritically, the language but

---

1. We do not condone the validity and the diagnostic use of *DSM-IV-TR,* but refer to it to provide a platform for person-centred theorists and practitioners to show that the work they do is of relevance to the wider mental health community.

above all the conceptual framework of the medical model (Sanders, 2005). There is of course a perfectly legitimate range of responses to working with other mental health professionals. (See, for example, Sanders, 2005, as opposed to Sommerbeck, 2005.) We can either choose to set ourselves against the prevailing orthodoxy, or find ways to work with it in a complementary fashion: with integrity. What we cannot do is sacrifice the foundational principles of the person-centred approach in order to accommodate the medical model uncritically.

All person-centred practitioners need to be clear about what marks out the genius of the approach. Neither Richard nor Stephen is prone to a ghetto mentality. We believe that there must be within the approach a broad-ranging and tolerant dialogue about those perspectives which range from the classical, client-centred model, through process-orientated and integrative models, to the experiential and focusing models. (See, for an introduction to these, and a pacific dialogue between them, Sanders 2004.) However, there are a number of baseline principles which mark out the radical nature of our approach, and which *of necessity* place us with our allies, the proponents of a positive and critical psychology (e.g., Maddux, Snyder and Lopez, 2004).

'HERE I STAND. I CAN DO NO OTHER'

With these words, Martin Luther divided medieval Europe in two: Catholic and Protestant. We must also be prepared to take a principled stance. Where do *we* stand? We want to suggest that there are a number of key principles which mark out the person-centred approach in particular in terms of psychopathology:

• The actualising tendency as a theoretical construct prompts us to see that even in great distress human beings have the ability to seek for themselves that which is growthful. In fact, the power of this tendency is such that clients have an irritating habit of using therapy in novel and creative ways, without due regard for theory! (See in particular Bohart and Tallman, 1999.) However, on some occasions, that which is actualised is imperfect, and in some degree dysfunctional.

• So-called symptoms are therefore not to be seen as failings of a system, but of the human organism's response to environmental or socio-psychological stress. This means that symptoms are too important to medicate away, for they abound with meaning. If they are not heard, they will continue to generate distressing experience. (See Garry Prouty on hallucinations, Chapter 15; also more generally, Bentall, 2004)

• Human existence is a complex interpenetration of the physical, the mental, the social and, some would say, the spiritual. Person-centred practice is of essence holistic. Therefore individuals in distress cannot be reduced to symptoms, or to the physical alone. The mind-brain is a system that exhibits a highly complex ongoing translation process between the biochemical and the meaning levels (Gray, 2004). The medical model tends to ignore or reduce to mere epiphenomena human meaning. It fails to see that the mind-brain correspondence is two-way: if the notion of meaning in life has any validity whatsoever. Meaning generates electrical, biochemical and morphological phenomena, as well as *vice versa*. The (at least) two levels implicit in the notion of mind-brain interpenetrate.

- The relief of distress depends on the establishment and inhabiting of psychological contact. Thus, even the severest distress—that which is often called psychosis, a loss of grip on everyday reality—is of essence a relational condition. People with psychosis above all need well-judged human relationships. These need not even be professional. Some of the most spectacular effects have been achieved by lay people in therapeutic communities, such as the Soteria Project (See Sanders, Chapter 16 this volume, pp. 194 –5). People with psychosis can be joyful and creative even when living with some level of distress and disorientation (Jamison, 1993).

- It is possible that the person-centred approach, even when it stands out against the medicalisation of distress, can collude in seeing therapy as symptom relief. Our clients, day by day, express appreciation when they 'feel better'. This is seductive. The positive psychology perspective is necessary to remind us that even in distress we can grow towards fulfilment. I draw attention to the last sentence of Chapter 5 in this volume: 'Maybe the gift that suffering offers us is the opportunity to live more tenderly in the world'.

- Therapy always happens in a particular context: the wealthy suburb in which meaninglessness is sedated by alcohol; the deprived city community in which environmental stress is endemic and, to some degree, seemingly intractable; the rural community in which personal wealth is often matched by communal deprivation. The causes of distress are thus communal, social and hence political and spiritual. The political aspect of person-centred therapy (Proctor et al., 2006) is part of its holistic approach. The medical model, by contrast, tends to be politically suffocating of human initiative. If drugs are all that is available, even if they bring some relief, this militates against wholeness of body, mind and society. These three cannot be separated.

Here we stand. We can do no other.

POSITIVE PSYCHOLOGY

> The single most important contribution of positive psychology has been to provide a collective identity—a common voice and language for researchers and practitioners from all persuasions who share an interest in health as well as in sickness—in the fulfilment of potential as well as the amelioration of pathology. (Linley and Joseph, 2004: 4)

On the surface, positive psychology takes an interest in well-being, in human happiness. It observes that psychology has been traditionally preoccupied with the pathological and, above all, with a deficit model of being human. The new focus upon well-being is welcome in itself. The movement toward well-being—or being fully-functioning to use the term employed by Carl Rogers—has always been the focus of person-centred

3

psychology, even when working with those who are deeply distressed (Joseph and Linley, 2006a). Here the person-centred approach and the positive psychology movement most obviously collide.

However, it is significant that, unlike person-centred psychology, positive psychology does not yet lay claim to any meta-theoretical position, and has perhaps unknowingly adopted the medical model, insofar as many of its proponents may view the facilitation of well-being as a separate task to that of the alleviation of psychopathology (Joseph and Linley, 2006b). Person-centred practitioners can learn from the positive psychology research literature—and the alignment of the person-centred community with the positive psychology movement might prove beneficial in combating the marginalisation of the person-centred approach, and bringing it back into the mainstream. But positive psychology can also learn from the meta-theoretical perspective of the person-centred approach to ground its thinking and research (Joseph and Linley, 2006a; Patterson and Joseph, 2007).

While there is much that academic psychology is coming to say about what makes humans contented and hence productive, the challenge to person-centred theory is different from this. Therapy deals largely, but not exclusively, with those who are distressed. A deficit model of distress might lead us to assume that relief is about a return to some state of contented normality, which, were it not for the causes of distress, the person would have inhabited all along. This seems a rather sentimental, unimaginative and inaccurate version of being human. Distress is part of the very fabric of our existence. In coming to dwell with it creatively, whether or not the apparent symptoms abate, the potential emerges of being more fulfilled in some sense than if the distress had been absent.

Positive psychology challenges person-centred therapists to hear that growth in themselves and their clients which comes from suffering (Joseph and Linley, 2006a). There may be a number of reasons for being reluctant to hear this. How is it to say to another 'You have suffered and have grown'? It may sound unempathic or even impudent. Even the person-centred practitioner can lapse into a deficit model of distress. Until we can hear that our clients grow precisely *because* they have suffered, then we will underestimate, and sell short, the human potential that we claim to facilitate. This book of case studies is a window upon such growth.

WHY CASE STUDIES?

On person-centred training courses, it is usual for the beginning counsellor to have to write a number of case studies, sometimes supported with audio- or video-tapes of sessions. This is intended to demonstrate that the would-be counsellor can show a rationale for her pattern of working and a detailed and critical understanding of why the therapy is effective. It is therefore ironic that there are relatively few case studies in person-centred literature. (I distinguish here a *case study*, in which the writer researches and learns, from a *vignette*, in which the writer simply makes a teaching point. We have written both—and they differ.)

4

Evidence-based practice in counselling and psychotherapy generally has a tendency to prefer that which can be measured. It is of course 'scientific' and 'proves' things. In fact, therapists learn from experience, validate their own work qualitatively and, by and large, show a set of assessment criteria which stem from an intelligent listening to complex experience (Daniel and McLeod, 2006). Psychotherapy is too human and too complex to reduce to outcome measures. (There are, however, outcome measures which are particularly congruent with the person-centred approach. See Patterson and Joseph, Chapter 17 this volume). To read a case study is to take on board, and be helped to think through at depth, the heart of therapy.

Within this book of case studies, the use of material that is rooted in reflective practice will be marked by the following characteristics:

- One practitioner, whether beginning or mature, can 'look over the shoulder' at another's work, engage humanely with it, and, by entering an internal dialogue with the work, grow in his or her own theory and practice.
- Theory will be rooted in practice, and practice in reflection. This is an essential aspect of the supervisory / consultative process which is an ethical imperative for counsellors.
- Case studies are also practitioner research, and so quite specific pieces of empirical evidence that the approach is effective with particular client groups. The empirical nature of this evidence complements the deductive nature of statements of theory and of quantitative outcome research.
- A number of case studies give voice, directly or indirectly, to the client's experience and appraisal of therapy. This is the sort of outcome measure that ought to matter.
- 'Just show me.' There are a number of interested parties in counselling and psychotherapy who are not professionally trained. The person-centred approach has not done a good job in commending itself to those who fund or manage therapy provision, particularly in the medical and statutory sectors. There is a cultural gulf to be overcome in this task. Case studies help those from outside the approach to understand what the approach is *really* about. It is therefore also useful for those who train or supervise across modalities.
- The theory of therapy is empirical. It comes from puzzlement. Why does this work? Why doesn't that? Case studies show the importance of the growing edge of person-centred theory. Margaret Warner's long-term study of Luke as a source of her conceptualisation about his process is paradigmatic of this. (See Chapter 13 this volume, and also Warner, 2002.)
- Therapy is above all about encounter at depth. Case studies, because they are human and empirical, allow this to be explored.
- Clients use therapy in unpredictable ways. There is, we suspect, much still to learn about this. Case studies bring out the client's creativity, sometimes in spite of the therapist's lack of imagination.
- Case studies demonstrate the social and political context of therapy. (See Chapters 5 and 16 in this volume.)
- Case studies demonstrate that, as the therapeutic process unfolds, changes that occur within the client in their thoughts and feelings—and in how they behave and relate

to the external world—are idiosyncratic, holistic, and directed toward finding meaning, gaining autonomy, relating to others—i.e., those aspects of well-being that we would characterise as fully functioning.

THE CONTENTS OF THIS BOOK

In *Person-Centred Psychopathology*, a range of essays was assembled in which theorists of international repute set out the basis for understanding how person-centred meta-theory addressed the questions, the raw facts of life, which in traditional psychology fall under the heading of psychopathology. In editing these essays, we came to appreciate the breadth and depth of engagement with these issues. Together, the thinking of some twenty individuals made an eloquent claim for the person-centred approach, understood as a positive psychological therapy, to be treated with the utmost seriousness.

In this volume, the focus moves from theory to practice, and thus to practitioner research and to evidence. It is important to practitioners, beginning therapists, therapist educators and supervisors, as well as those who oversee and fund the practice of therapy, that our approach is effective. The case studies challenge the current myths that the person-centred approach is nothing more than counselling for the worried well; that effective psychological treatment requires specific diagnosis and evidence, after the style of the medical model; that distress is an illness to be cured rather than a human condition through which people have the innate capacity to grow.

The first volume sets out the philosophy which roots the approach, while this volume describes and thus evidences the modes of practice which stem from this philosophy. It is not essential to have read *Person-Centred Psychopathology* to benefit from this volume, but to have done so is useful.

The first volume began with Catherine Clarke's account of her experience as a user of mental health services. This second volume begins with a parallel account of Alex Payne's experience of being a trainee clinical psychologist. She makes a cogent case for facing her internal incongruence in being compelled to act as a diagnostician, for seeing and coming to believe in the essential resourcefulness of her clients and for the need to overcome cultural conditioning in order to move away from the power dynamics of the medical model and of western patriarchy in general.

The next three case studies in this volume crucially represent the voice of the client. Those forms of treatment of mental distress which objectify the sufferer and reduce emotional pain and growth to mere symptoms need to confront the actual experience of those who seek help. Indeed, clients have knack of using therapy which defies most theoretical constructs, save that of the actualising tendency (Bohart and Tallman, 1999). Matthew Campling offers a first-hand account of his anorexia. He demonstrates that one configuration has had the ability to keep the rest of him safe. He reflects on links between his own experience as a client and his growing experience as a therapist. Next, Gillian Proctor, together with Ann Regan, maps out the key motifs in Ann's work in therapy. Because of the process of meeting at the end of therapy to review perspectives, Ann's view of her therapy has a unique voice. It not only adds confirmation to the power of the therapeutic conditions, but also demonstrates, in Gillian's words, the need of therapists to find confirmation (or otherwise) of their work in their client's genuine experience. This is practitioner research. Tracey Sanders' and June O'Brien's account of their work together not only offers another version of a client's experience and of a therapist's conceptualisation of this, but also constitutes a major plea that therapists should work in particular with those who are socially disadvantaged, and should voluntarily quit the ghetto of the well-to-do. This chapter creatively echoes Pete Sanders' plea (Chapter 16, this volume) to take seriously the socio-political context of therapy.

There follow eight case studies on particular themes and perspectives. Elaine Catterall writes about what is, ostensibly, post-natal depression. However, it is also about the significance of the environment and, hence, of the politics of therapy. She demonstrates that when there is no cure available, just because there can be no immediate shift in environmental pressures, then the person-centred approach—seen as the implementation of positive psychology—has the capacity to render meaningful the painful in a client's life precisely through the act of relating at depth. Jerold Bozarth then describes a dialogue between Ann Glauser, the therapist, Berdie, her client, and himself as Ann's supervisor, who undertook an in-depth interview with both therapist and client to explore what had facilitated client growth.

Jan Hawkins explores her work with a client who, as a result of childhood sexual abuse, experiences dissociative processing. Jan's chapter illustrates just why diagnosis is counter-productive—while being guided by the client is so potent. The subject of Jan's reflection is, of course, not really dissociative processing, but a human being who is in relationship with her. We see how the dissociated elements of the client, while at times distressing, are also highly functional in defending the client. Jan relates to each element. The work is also a tribute to the everyday love which therapists feel for clients and clients for therapists. Richard Worsley then explores the stuckness of chronic depression and the role of diagnosis in perpetuating this, since some clients take great comfort in being diagnosed. This is a challenge to the role of congruent responding in the therapist. Again, the focus is upon the need to conceptualise how psychological pain can bring about growth, and overcome the passivity induced by medical model formulations. Watch out for the sting in the tail of this chapter. Always read your 'thank you' cards with care!

It could be said that Jerold Bozarth and Richard Worsley are making contradictory points. The former argues that the paramount task is to make space for the client to guide the therapy; the latter argues that there are times when it is crucial that the therapist congruently opposes him or herself to elements of the client's awareness. It would be naïve to see this as a disagreement, or even as typical of the differences between classical and experiential therapy. The two cases witness to the complexity of relating. There are two metaphors for relating: accompanying and being face to face. The mature therapist aims at discernment between these two in response to the client's whole being—expressed and unexpressed.

Martin van Kalmthout explores the case of Hans Sievez. This is an unusual and intriguing piece of work. Ostensibly it argues that the mature therapist can both work hard to conceptualise the direction of therapy—and the therapist's hopes, aims and intentions within that—while at the same times experiencing therapy as unpredictable and creative, thus knowing the necessary freedom to practise. However, van Kalmthout also shows how important is the life of imagination for continued professional development; for Sievez is the subject of the Dutch novel, *Kneeling on a Bed of Violets*. The novel focuses upon the disabling pressures experienced by Sievez from within a Christian sect, so it is also a discussion of the possibility of thinking through what is functional and dysfunctional in issues of spirituality. This is an area of life that many therapists feel ill-equipped to enter. Van Kalmthout offers us a way of thinking about the possibility of working in this area.

The next three case studies, each and together, demonstrate that mature, person-centred therapy, together with pre-therapy, as developed by Garry Prouty, permit work with those clients who have impaired contact with the phenomenal world: those often termed psychotic. The first is a conversation between Barbara Krietemeyer—in her work to establish psychological contact with a client who is 'deeply regressed, mentally retarded and psychotic'—and Garry Prouty, who developed the procedures that Barbara is engaging. Here is a chapter which is both deeply practical and reflective. There follows Dion van Werde's account of his work with Henry. This also illustrates the application of Prouty's pre-therapy. However, the reader might notice a very different feel— particular, I suspect, to the author—and the impact again of context. Van Werde is working on a hospital ward. He focuses long-term not merely upon function and dysfunction in individuals but also upon function and dysfunction in mental health organisations. The point he makes about Henry, though, I offer in his own words; 'The hypothesis of Pre-Therapy—that contact and symptomatic functioning are inversely connected—appears plausible and proven'.

Margaret Warner offers us further thoughts upon her client, Luke, who exhibits a schizophrenic thought disorder. This chapter witnesses Warner's dogged commitment to thinking through time and again her learning from one client. (See Warner, 2002, for an earlier stage in this process of reflection.) She demonstrates how reflective practice allows the development of a phenomenology of a particular disorder which is both humane and unique to the client, and which is capable of useful generalisation. This stands in marked contrast to the impersonal nature of endless taxonomies of mental illness. Luke is Thou, not It.

The last four chapters before the Conclusion show, together, how case study and reflective practice generate new theory and new research. Brian Levitt offers a scholarly review of unpublished casework by Carl Rogers: the case of Gina. The chapter demonstrates the power of a willingness on Rogers' part not to direct the client. However, it also shows the fact that the positive psychology perspective was inherent in Rogers' work from early days. Gina talks of her fear. At the end of the session she still feels fear but her relationship to it has changed. Although fear is painful, Gina grows through it.

In the next chapter, Garry Prouty takes up Van Werde's theme of psychotic hallucination. He then develops a profound theoretical framework for this phenomenon, based on the concept of pre-symbolic expression and illustrated from three phases of therapy with a client. From this, it becomes experientially clear to the reader that psychosis is deeply imbued with meaning, if only the therapist can learn to hear and respond appropriately. Next, Pete Sanders uses a brief case study to take forward his argument from the previous volume against the medicalisation of distress (Joseph and Worsley, 2005, Chapter 3). This is a clarion call to take seriously the socio-political implications of the person-centred approach, and a useful taster of the fuller argument of Proctor et al., (2006). The concluding chapter takes us back to the task of the person-centred approach to demonstrate our credentials in evidence-based practice. Thomas Patterson and Stephen Joseph offer a detailed account of those instruments which measure outcomes of therapy, in ways congruent with the person-centred theories of personality and therapy, to show how empirical research need not be grounded in medical model ideology.

CONFIDENTIALITY

Throughout, material has been anonymised, except in those three cases in which the name of the client or supervisee is included because they have co-authored the chapter. In all other cases, individual authors hold evidence of informed consent from their clients. Time and again authors are struck by the generous willingness of clients to participate as co-researchers. This is not only moving but also a challenge to the acquiring of truly informed consent. Obtaining consent echoes issues around conditions of worth, conformity and, thus, the potential power imbalance of any therapeutic relationship.

However, the work involved in just making a start on writing up a case study can also add greatly to the therapeutic relationship. The process of negotiation and of writing, if worked out within a person-centred relationship of integrity, itself constitutes a seeking in retrospect for a shared understanding of the therapeutic experience within the client-therapist dyad. When, in writing up the case of Hilary (Worsley, 2002, Chapter 13), Richard invited her to read through the final account—as he thought it to be—Hilary not only asked for some amendments, as expected, but took the paper to her younger sister. The two sisters then instigated some informal family therapy between them. In the paper each recognised the deep incongruences which bedevilled the family network. Love and relating deepened.

Our thanks are due, above all, to our clients, those represented in this book and those many thousands of others who have taught us the profound lesson of what it is to be human.

REFERENCES

American Psychiatric Association (2000) *Diagnostic and Statistical Manual of Mental Disorders–IV–TR*. Arlington VA: American Psychiatric Publishing. (Cited as *DSM–IV–TR*.)

Bentall, RP (2004) *Madness Explained: Psychosis and human nature*. London: Penguin.

Bohart, AC and Tallman, K (1999) *How Clients Make Therapy Work: The process of active self-healing*. Washington: American Psychological Association.

Daniel, T and McLeod, J (2006) Weighing up the evidence: A qualitative analysis of how person-centred counsellors evaluate the effectiveness of their practice. *Counselling and Psychotherapy Research, 6*, 244–9.

Gray, J (2004) *Consciousness: Creeping up on the hard problem*. Oxford: Oxford University Press.

Jamison, KR (1993) *Touched with Fire: Manic-depressive illness and the artistic temperament*. New York: Free Press Paperbacks.

Joseph, S and Linley PA (2006a) *Positive Therapy: a meta-theory for positive psychological practice*. London: Routledge.

Joseph, S and Linley, PA (2006b) Positive psychology versus the medical model? *American Psychologist, 61*, 332–3.

Joseph, S and Worsley, R (eds) (2005) *Person-Centred Psychopathology: A positive psychology of mental health*. Ross-on-Wye: PCCS Books.

Linley, PA and Joseph, S (eds) (2004) *Positive Psychology in Practice*. New York: John Wiley.

Maddux, JE, Snyder, CR and Lopez, SJ (2004) Toward a positive clinical psychology: Deconstructing the illness ideology and constructing an ideology of human strengths and potential. In PA Linley and S Joseph (eds) *Positive Psychology in Practice* (pp. 320–34). Hoboken, NJ: Wiley.

Patterson, TG and Joseph, S (2007) Person-centered personality theory: Support from self-determination theory and positive psychology. *Journal of Humanistic Psychology, 47*, 117–39.

Proctor, G, Cooper, M, Sanders, P and Malcolm, B (eds) (2006) *Politicizing the Person-Centred Approach: An agenda for social change*. Ross-on-Wye: PCCS Books.

Sanders, P (ed) (2004) *Tribes of the Person-Centred Nation: An introduction to the schools of therapy related to the person-centred approach*. Ross-on-Wye: PCCS Books.

Sanders, P (2005) Principled and strategic opposition to the medicalisation of distress and all of its apparatus. In S Joseph and R Worsley (eds), *Person-Centred Psychopathology: A positive psychology of mental health* (pp. 21–42). Ross-on-Wye: PCCS Books.

Sommerbeck, L (2005) The complementarity between client-centred therapy and psychiatry: The theory and the practice. In S Joseph and R Worsley (eds), *Person-Centred Psychopathology: A positive psychology of mental health* (pp. 110–27). Ross-on-Wye: PCCS Books.

Warner, MS (2002) Luke's dilemmas: A client-centered / experiential model of processing with a schizophrenic thought disorder. In JC Watson, RN Goldman and MS Warner (eds) *Client-Centered and Experiential Psychotherapy in the 21st Century: Advances in theory, research and practice*. Ross-on-Wye: PCCS Books.

Worsley, R (2002) *Process Work in Person-Centred Therapy: Phenomenological and existential perspectives*. Basingstoke: Palgrave.

CHAPTER 2

COMING FULL CIRCLE: ADOPTING AND RELINQUISHING THE EXPERT STANCE AS A CLINICAL PSYCHOLOGIST

ALEX PAYNE

This chapter describes my journey through clinical psychology training and the circumstances through which I came to adopt, and then relinquish, the expert role in my work with clients. In doing so, I will provide information regarding my background prior to embarking on clinical training; my expectations of the role of a clinical psychologist; my experience of the first month of training; the adoption of the expert role through the first and second year of training; the watershed that occurred in my final year of training that was the relinquishing of the role of expert and the coinciding adoption of a client-centred approach. In describing the relinquishing of the role of expert, I will discuss clinical examples of using a client-centred approach that I felt helped to cement my belief in the approach. I will also provide clinical examples of clinicians adopting the expert role with outcomes, which I considered to be potentially damaging to the client. I will then discuss why I think clinical psychologists are sometimes reluctant to relinquish the expert role and adopt a client-centred approach.

PERSONAL BACKGROUND

My enthusiasm for psychology was sparked during my A levels. During this time I learned about a number of famous studies, which gave me an interest in understanding more about human behaviour. Following this I undertook an applied psychology undergraduate degree hoping that it would give me further understanding of human behaviour and a job working within the field. During the third year of the degree I was required to undertake a clinical placement to gain insight into the application of psychology within the workplace. I chose to work as an Assistant Psychologist at a medium-secure psychiatric hospital. Being unqualified, my role did not involve therapy with clients. Instead I co-facilitated group therapy, which was largely predetermined in the form of sessions. The sessions were primarily psychoeducational and I did not hear much about clients' experiences. Similarly, any work I undertook on an individual basis with clients was manualised and psychoeducational, involving teaching clients about drugs or enhancing problem-solving strategies. I worked alongside clinical psychologists and viewed them as very powerful and important; however, their work with clients was never discussed with me and remained elusive yet intriguing. Having gained a little insight into the applied role of the clinical psychologist I decided that this was the avenue I wanted to pursue.

I completed my degree and was offered the opportunity to commence a PhD in developmental psychology, which I accepted. I chose to study factors associated with the development of conduct problems in school-age children and was delighted to be able to conduct research into something I was passionate about, especially thinking that I might be able to make a difference to the people involved. This research experience was invaluable in terms of equipping me with the skills to conduct exciting and innovative research, yet it did not equip me with the therapeutic skills required to work as a clinical psychologist. I felt that although research was important to me, I was lacking that connection with clients that I had originally wanted. That was when I realised that my heart was really with working directly with people and that the clinical psychology training route was my passion. I was fortunate enough to secure a place on a clinical psychology training course, which commenced immediately following my PhD.

EXPECTATIONS OF THE ROLE OF THE CLINICAL PSYCHOLOGIST

At the time of starting the clinical psychology training, my understanding of the role of the clinical psychologist was one of a person who worked with a variety of client groups and mental health difficulties, providing a range of therapeutic techniques, conducting psychometric assessments, writing reports and collaborating with other health professionals in determining client care. I thought of the clinical psychologist as someone who worked predominantly from a medical model; someone who took referrals from the GP and applied various treatments based on the client's 'diagnosis'. I assumed that the clinical psychologist spent hours poring over relevant literature to find answers to clients' problems and using the information to help clients gain mastery over their difficulties. I suppose in that respect I assumed that the clinical psychologist was the expert within the therapeutic relationship, but at that time I did not consider that I would adopt that stance. With no experience of sitting in a room with a client and asking them about their difficulties, I never thought of myself as being an expert. I felt very incompetent in comparison to my peers on the course, who appeared to have plenty of clinical experience and therapeutic skills. I felt that my best way forward was to come alongside clients in helping them make sense of how, why, where and when difficulties arose and how best they might manage them.

THE FIRST MONTH OF TRAINING

The first month of training was, for me, a rich mixture of experiences and emotions. The focus was on being with a client and gaining an understanding of what the difficulties were, and generally conducting a basic assessment. A lot of time was spent learning about and practising reflecting back to clients, paraphrasing, empathising and summarising. We were taught to just sit with the client and not offer advice, as this was to come later in the teaching block. We were informed that these therapeutic skills were the basic therapeutic elements as outlined by Rogers (1951), and that if we could master these we were ready to learn about other interventions such as cognitive-behavioural and psychodynamic techniques. By the end of the first month of teaching I felt I had learnt about Rogers' core conditions and was ready to move on to learning the techniques that would differentiate me from other health professionals in terms of being able to treat mental illness.

ADOPTION OF THE EXPERT STANCE THROUGHOUT THE FIRST TWO YEARS OF TRAINING

Alongside clinical placements throughout the first and second years of training, the course also provided teaching on various psychotherapeutic approaches. Predominantly we were taught cognitive-behavioural and psychodynamic approaches and techniques to help clients understand how and why their difficulties arose, what was maintaining them and how to intervene to alleviate distress.

The cognitive-behavioural teaching component taught us how to identify 'hot' thoughts and 'dysfunctional assumptions' and how to challenge clients' perception of events and ways of thinking about themselves and the world. Following teaching of generic cognitive-behavioural skills, we were then taught about specific cognitive-behavioural approaches to treating different disorders. I dutifully bought books outlining cognitive-behavioural interventions for a number of different emotional difficulties and used these to inform my practice with clients while on clinical placements. At the time, it felt as though these books were my saving grace because I was able to read the GP referral or assessment report and identify the diagnosis the client had been given. I could then go to the shelf, pick up the relevant book and spend time reading about specific techniques to intervene with the client's problems. Being very new to working with clients in a therapeutic setting, these books were like my safety net. They enabled me to present myself as knowing more about the clients' difficulties than they did, and this helped me to feel like the expert in the relationship.

Similarly, the psychodynamic teaching component taught us how to formulate client difficulties and use the formulation to generate hypotheses regarding what might be underlying client difficulties. It was assumed that clients would be largely unaware of the 'true' cause of their problems and that, as therapists, we could make interpretations of clients' dialogue to highlight the unconscious elements of distress to them. Again, I bought books to help me understand the approach in more depth and to guide me in my clinical work. This approach felt far more unstructured than the cognitive-behavioural approach and I felt less certain of what I was supposed to be doing. It felt more like I was trying to make sense of client experiences and making judgements as to what might be creating distress and feeding it back to clients. I was slightly more comfortable with this approach since it enabled some flexibility in what clients chose to accept or not. It felt more collaborative and less predetermined than cognitive-behavioural therapy and I was relieved that it enabled much deeper exploration of clients' problems. I also felt clients were generally more receptive to this approach and that it was much more collaborative than cognitive-behavioural approaches.

As time passed I became more comfortable working in these ways and felt my competence increasing. I felt I was making a positive difference to the majority of the clients that I saw. There were a few clients with whom I did not feel I had developed a good therapeutic relationship and I felt frustrated that, sometimes, no matter how much I tried to help, they seemed unreceptive to my suggestions. I even tried switching between cognitive-behavioural and psychodynamic approaches with some of these clients in the hope that something, somewhere, would 'fit' for them and would be helpful.

In conversations with my peers on the course I became aware that I was working in the same way they were and had the same understanding of the approaches. Other trainees had difficulties with some clients and so I thought this was just the norm and attributed these difficulties to clients not being 'psychologically minded'. I had no doubt that I was trying my best for clients and, although I did not feel as though I was an extremely competent and experienced practitioner, I by no means thought that I was not capable of being a clinical psychologist. Supervisors had never given me negative feedback about my work with clients and I had no reason to believe I was doing anything 'wrong'. I entered the third year thinking that I had gained a variety of experience working with a range of client difficulties and that I could continue to be of help and learn much more.

For my final year placements I chose to spend a year working within two settings. The first setting was a forensic service for clients with learning disabilities while the second specialised in working with trauma victims. I chose these placements because I felt that the core placements had given me the fundamental skills to work with clients with mainstream mental health difficulties, and that these specialised placements would provide me with the skills to work with highly complex and challenging difficulties. I thought that these placements would really make me the 'expert' since I would gain skills that other trainees would not have had the chance to develop. Little did I think that defining experiences during the third year would lead to a radical renouncing of the role of the expert and the adoption of an approach I had learnt so little about. I started work assuming that I would be capable of working effectively with these clients. This belief was severely challenged within the first few months of starting work in this field. My belief about my expertise was shattered through listening to traumatic stories, and through trying to help people overcome traumatic experiences.

On my first day at the trauma service I answered the telephone to a woman who could only be described as being in complete turmoil. She was so distressed her speech was barely coherent and her thoughts switched from one trauma to another in a matter of seconds. I found it very difficult to concentrate on what she was saying and extremely difficult to comprehend the extent of the traumas she had experienced. I had never heard anything like it. The woman remained on the telephone for over an hour and yet within minutes I felt completely powerless and totally ineffectual as a therapist. I did not know what to say, and felt as though all the skills I would normally have drawn upon were inappropriate. Given the number of traumas the woman had experienced, her beliefs about the world as an unsafe and unfair place seemed rational. Given the extent of her turmoil, her beliefs about being unable to cope with life seemed valid and understandable. I was at a loss as to what to say and left my first day in the job feeling as though I was certainly no expert.

As time went by I increasingly came across this situation. It felt as though nothing I said or did made a difference. I seriously started to doubt my expertise. I defended these feelings of incompetence by telling myself that clients were to blame for their difficulties and that they did not really want to help themselves. I found myself becoming increasingly anxious and low about my ability to make a difference for these people. This was not helpful for my clients. I knew I was unable to remain anxious and low and decided that it was imperative for my self-esteem and the well-being of the clients that I found a way of working with them that would truly meet their needs. Consequently, I started to immerse myself in the client-centred approach and was amazed at the difference it made to these clients to be truly listened to, understood and to have their experiences validated.

Previously I had employed psychological approaches that set me up as the expert on the clients' lives, giving them advice and making suggestions as to how they should think and behave. The experience of feeling powerless to help these traumatised clients made me step back and think about what it was I was trying to do and why it was not working as well as it had with previous clients. I was disgusted at the way in which I had imposed my ideas on clients in the past and had not trusted them to heal themselves. I had inadvertently made those clients reliant upon me to provide them with the answers to their difficulties, and in doing so had stifled their inherent ability to heal themselves. In addition, I suddenly realised why I had experienced extreme frustration with some clients who did not respond to the cognitive-behavioural or psychodynamic approaches I had been using. The reality was that I was not listening to them. I had preconceived ideas of what their difficulties were and what was the best way of managing them. This did not leave any room for clients to express their own ideas, and my adoption of the expert role very likely led to them feeling unable to say when they felt I was completely off the mark. The guilt I experienced in realising this led to a drastic change in the way I worked with clients from then on.

PUTTING THE CLIENT-CENTRED APPROACH INTO PRACTICE

After embracing the client-centred approach it was time to try putting it into practice. Coincidentally, my first experience of this happened to involve the woman to whom I had first answered the telephone. In circumstances similar to our first exchange, she was in turmoil and had started to shout at me in desperation. She was shouting at me to help her and tell her what to do. I remained quiet. My mind was giving me lots of options that would have offered a very superficial and short-lived means of reducing her anxiety and I felt that it was unethical to make such suggestions. After a period of silence she shouted at me, 'Why aren't you helping me?' I was petrified to answer honestly but felt I had to be truthful. I commented, 'Because I don't know what to say. You've had so many traumatic things happen to you that I can't make it better for you. I could give you some suggestions but they are unlikely to help you and I really don't know what to say.' There was a long pause and I was frightened that I had been completely unprofessional. She very calmly said, 'Thank you. That's the first time anyone has been honest with me. It really helps that you believe me.' Without saying goodbye she hung up the telephone.

I have never forgotten that conversation because it was the first time that I did not try and provide a solution or act as the expert and, contrary to my prior expectations, it had a beneficial effect. I realised that clients with long-standing histories of interpersonal violence and abuse are unlikely to have genuinely been heard, understood, believed, and more importantly trusted to be the experts on their own lives and able to heal themselves. This incident shifted my beliefs again. I no longer felt totally incompetent. In fact I felt more competent and empowered to help because now I had a new philosophy to work with that I felt was, ethically, much more acceptable than the prescriptive approaches I had used previously. I realised that I do not always need to be able to provide the answers and, indeed, it is unethical to do so. I am gradually regaining my confidence as a therapist and my belief that I am able to help victims of interpersonal violence. More importantly, I strongly believe that in order to be a competent therapist it is essential to believe that clients can heal themselves, given the appropriate conditions.

Since that first moment of realisation of how beneficial the client-centred approach can be, I have had many more experiences of working in this way that have really benefited the client in ways that, I believe, prescriptive approaches might not have. I worked in a medium-secure setting with a young woman who had resided there for six years. Although she had made tremendous progress in terms of understanding and managing her distress she referred herself to psychology services. I met with her and, from the first moment, I made it clear that discussions in therapy were going to be entirely determined by her. She chose to speak with me regarding issues of loss and abuse. For the first couple of months that we met, she would tell me a little about her experiences and intersperse this with conversations about totally unrelated topics. Had I been working within a different psychotherapeutic orientation I might have stated to her that, although it was difficult, it was necessary that I heard the details in order to make sense of what she had been through. In helping her make sense of her traumas from a cognitive-behavioural perspective I might have insisted that she relive the experiences in order to process them adequately. I did neither of these things and, in hindsight, I think it would have destroyed the trust we had built up and resulted in her terminating therapy. Instead, I spent time talking with her about whatever she chose with equal interest. I think she was probably dipping in and out of discussing painful material with me in order to manage her distress.

After a few months the same client came to a session in quite a distressed state. She informed me that she did not think that talking about her issues of loss and abuse was helping her and, in fact she felt it was making her feel lower. I acknowledged and accepted her ability to know what was best for her and asked her what she would like to use the sessions for. She stated that she had decided that she could not change the past and therefore she would like to focus on making a positive future for herself. During the sessions we discussed her strengths and what she would like for the future. Occasionally she would briefly revert back to talking about her experiences of loss and abuse and I did not resist this. I felt that she inherently knew what was best for her and followed her lead. As the months passed she became much brighter and more positive about her future. I accepted that there were times she did not feel able to meet with me and did not threaten her with terminating therapy as other therapists might have done. I felt that we had a very good therapeutic relationship and that she was able to trust me. I felt that accepting her unconditionally, being congruent, validating her experiences and trusting her to know what was best for herself was far more therapeutic than any prescriptive approach would have been. This experience bolstered my confidence in the client-centred approach and my belief that you do not have to be directive in order to help a client.

Another experience that increased my belief in trusting clients to know what is best for themselves happened while working for a charitable organisation. A client that regularly used the drop-in service and attended group therapy called one day stating that she did not feel able to attend as she felt 'risky'. The manager of the service was away and the client felt that she might 'do something stupid' if she came and felt unsafe without the manager's presence. The staff member who answered the phone reassured the client that it would be fine, that the staff would be able to manage any situation that arose and that the client should attend. The staff member was acting out of kindness and trying to make the client feel cared for and supported and I have no doubt that she thought she was doing the best for the client. What happened next was very unfortunate and a strong reminder for me that we should trust clients' judgements of what they can and cannot tolerate.

The client attended the centre feeling very anxious and afraid. After the group, other clients had left the building and only two female members of staff remained. They were busy and the client was left alone. Becoming increasingly anxious and distressed, the client started self-harming. The members of staff tried approaching her but this made her more afraid and she started threatening them with the razor she was using to self-harm. Not knowing what to do the members of staff locked themselves in an office and called the police. Before the police arrived, the client fled the building, frightened, anxious and with a weapon in her possession. I was informed of the incident shortly afterwards and an emergency staff meeting was held to decide what to do. The majority of staff favoured banning the client from attending the services again. I was shocked, disgusted and outraged that this client had originally called stating that she felt unsafe and did not want to attend, yet was encouraged to attend anyway and was punished for not being able to manage—an outcome which she had predicted and warned staff about. Clearly she knew what was best for her that day, but one staff member's sense of knowing better created a distressing situation that need not have happened and that ultimately resulted in the client being punished and abused again.

Since relinquishing the role of the expert I have been shocked by the number of times I have witnessed clinical psychologists adopting the role of expert to the potential detriment of the client. A colleague and I ran a client-centred group therapy for clients with experiences of interpersonal violence. After presenting the findings of the group to other mental health professionals in the locality we were asked by a clinical psychologist about clients' capacity to tolerate listening to others' experiences of abuse. It was true that some clients found it more distressing than others but clients were aware that attendance at the group was their choice and these particular clients attended less regularly than others. The clinical psychologist asking the question seemed somewhat concerned about running such a group and the potential damage that might be done to the more distressed clients. He informed us that he had recently met with a client who had come seeking help in working through her experiences of abuse. He informed us that following the assessment he was very concerned that the client was still living in the home in which the abuse occurred and that he was worried that she would not be able to cope if he started discussing her experiences with her. Consequently, he suggested to her that she was not ready for therapy and she was not permitted to commence therapy. I felt that this action epitomised this role of the therapist as the 'expert'. This client had come seeking help and therefore was giving a clear message that she wished to embark on making sense of her experiences. How could the clinical psychologist have known better than the client how ready she was or how able she would be to manage? I highlighted to him that this client was living with these experiences every day and was managing them as best she could. Surely refusing her the right to therapy was another abusive act. We cannot mind-read and we cannot predict the future, so how can we possibly begin to dictate to clients what they are, or are not, capable of managing? Instead of making these judgements for clients, should we not be aligning ourselves alongside clients on the journey of making sense of experiences and supporting them through it? I am sure that it would become evident if clients were not coping, in which case either they would tell us, or we could reflect our own observations and allow clients to make their own decisions about continuing therapy. What will happen to this woman if every clinical psychologist she sees says she is not ready for therapy? I advocate client choice and I wonder why, seemingly, so many other clinical psychologists are reluctant to let go of the role of expert in the therapeutic relationship.

RELUCTANT TO CONSIDER RELINQUISHING THE ROLE OF THE EXPERT

Becoming a clinical psychologist is a long and arduous process. First, there is the undergraduate degree to complete, then a number of years working as an assistant psychologist on a low wage, or a number of years conducting research, or completing various other qualifications. Having managed to scale these hurdles, getting onto the training courses is no mean feat. The number of people grappling for training places far outweighs the number of places available. Many trainees experience multiple rejections before successfully securing a place. In addition to this, the ultimate achievement is that, upon obtaining the qualification, clinical psychologists get to call themselves 'Doctor', which in Western society is a position that is very highly regarded. This title portrays to people that the individual has undertaken years of training and is therefore the expert.

I am in no way suggesting that after years of training, requiring sheer determination, blood, sweat and tears, that the title of 'Doctor' is not warranted; far from it. I am suggesting that, because of how long it takes to train and how much experience is gained along the way, to consider oneself an expert would not be unusual. However, I think there is a vast difference between being an expert in neurosurgery or structural engineering and considering oneself an expert on someone else's thoughts, feelings and experiences. Given that everyone's experiences are so unique, is it ever possible to know or predict accurately how the individual will respond to, or manage, certain situations?

Had I not undertaken those final year placements, my knowledge of working in a client-centred way would have consisted of thinking that reflecting, empathising and summarising client's difficulties *for* them was what being client-centred entailed. I had no idea about Rogers' (1951) thoughts about the organismic valuing process and the actualising tendency and I certainly would never have considered trusting clients to know what was best for them. I guess looking back I would have questioned whether clients who knew what was best for themselves would be requesting professional assistance in resolving problems. What I had not accounted for was the impact of environmental influences in dictating client distress. I would never have thought that by providing Rogers' (1959) conditions of unconditional positive regard, congruence and empathy, clients would be offered the space to realise for themselves what would be best in alleviating distress.

My understanding at that time was that by empathising, actively listening, reflecting back and summarising I was being client-centred. Why would I only want to do that when I could also implement many of the cognitive-behavioural and psychodynamic techniques that I had spent so long learning? This is the response I often received from peers on the training course when I attempted to advocate a client-centred approach. 'I'm already doing it,' was the most frequent response.

I think the teaching of the client-centred approach was very misleading and trivialised by the training course. Having spent much time looking into this way of working I now understand that the approach is so much more than those very basic counselling skills. I think this might be one reason why clinical psychologists perceive the client-centred approach as very limited and not sufficient to help people without adding in techniques from other psychotherapeutic orientations. I think another reason might be that, having spent so long learning ways of 'treating' people, there is a reluctance to put those techniques to one side and never use them again. I also think that, perhaps to some clinical psychologists, to relinquish the role of expert, having spent so many years training to become one, seems nonsensical and insulting. I would argue that it does not take an expert to read chapters, aimed at addressing specific difficulties in a very specific way, and apply them within therapy sessions. Surely if clients had access to this information they would do it themselves, without years of training or considering themselves experts.

I think professionalism is demonstrated by being able to sit with a client through their distress and by believing in their ability to heal themselves. It takes professionalism to *not* give advice on anxiety management techniques and the like—which might make the client feel better temporarily but does not address underlying difficulties or provide space for psychological growth. It takes professionalism to truly empathise with a client, accept them unconditionally and to remain congruent: skills that for me are still very much in their infancy, but which I hope will continue to grow every day in my role as a clinical psychologist.

REFERENCE

Rogers, CR (1951) *Client-Centered Therapy*. London: Constable.

Rogers, CR (1959) A theory of therapy, personality and interpersonal relationships as developed in the client-centered framework. In S Koch (ed) *Psychology: The Study of a Science, Vol. 3.* (pp. 184–256). New York: McGraw-Hill.

CHAPTER 3

A PERSON-CENTRED RESPONSE TO EATING DISORDERS: A PERSONAL EXPERIENCE

MATTHEW CAMPLING

I have a particular, personal, reason for believing in the effectiveness of the client-centred approach. I developed anorexia in my late teens. Living in Durban, South Africa, in the mid-1970s there was no network of trained, supportive professionals. If I had not found a way to work through my illness myself and to recover from it, I would possibly have died or been forced into the nightmare world of the psychiatric ward. But, as it was, with a minimal degree of outside support, I discovered my own inner resources. A key aspect of my recovery was in rediscovering the joy of living: as the desire to survive and be healthy grew stronger, the anorexic self naturally became weaker and less able to dictate unreasonable behaviour.

Even though there is a much greater awareness of the existence of eating disorders now, there still seems to be a great deal of misinformation, and worse, about the illness. Therefore, I am writing about my own experience to offer a client's view of the nature of eating disorders and also to offer an alternative way to work with the client so they can actively cure themselves.

I write this chapter as a result of writing an article in *Therapy Today*, the journal of the British Association for Counselling and Psychotherapy (Campling, 2006). My writing that article came from a desire to be a different voice in the welter of confused and confusing babble surrounding the illness. When I heard, on television, the presenter of a 'problem' programme earnestly telling a young anorexic woman to 'remember, men like women with curves' I boiled. When a woman running a course on eating disorders complacently informed the group, 'I only work with anorexics and bulimics if they promise to eat properly,' I was aghast.

Both views fundamentally misunderstand the nature of the illness and the position of the person with an eating disorder. In simple, client-centred terms we need to be aware of the vital importance of *the internal locus of valuation* over the *external locus* which is represented in both the comments above (Mearns and Thorne, 1999: 10–12, 49–50).

To explain my experience of an eating disorder I need to go right back to childhood. For me, growing up in South Africa under apartheid was an ongoing, overwhelming, grief. I was a fat child, eating for stimulation and comfort. As I became interested in sex in my mid teens I decided to do something about the flabbiness I still felt. At that time I weighed about one hundred and fifty pounds on a 5'8" frame. I started dieting—not eating potatoes, drinking milk or snacking between meals—and began exercising.

We—my parents, two brothers and a sister—were living in a rural area outside Durban with a rather handy, immediate environment of hills and dales. I started by running downhill and walking up. I still remember the feeling of triumph, of being in control, that first day I could also run up hill. The weight began to drop off. I started to enjoy looking at my naked body in a mirror. At the same time, developing in a parallel way to the positive aspect of the dieting and exercise, the anorexic aspect was also beginning to gain strength. Because I did not have a cut-off point and extremes of behaviour were easy for me, losing another five—then ten—pounds became my sole aim.

I bought books on nutrition and learned the calorific value of every kind of food. I bought a book on Air Force exercises and would begin and end each day with a twenty-minute routine. At the same time, food stopped being my comfort and became my enemy. The anorexic voice began to speak: eating food was bad. Eating food was the cause of all my previous unhappiness. Therefore at the end of each day I would reward myself if I had denied myself food and punish myself (with reminders of how unacceptable to others being fat was) if I had given in.

At this point, about a year into the situation, people were noticing how thin I had become. My mother was helpful—she was the only person who offered sympathetic support. My two brothers' entirely unhelpful comment was that I looked like something out of Belsen. (At the time I found this comparison to the concentration camp experience upsetting. I believe the only way one can make a reference like this is with the greatest respect and responsibility towards the victims of the Holocaust and I include it only to show the impact my situation had on the family. At the time I thought my brothers were just being nasty but, in retrospect, I can understand that they were, in a clumsy way, genuinely expressing a response to my emaciated state).

There is so much that goes into the emotional world of someone with an eating disorder that if I commented on every aspect this chapter would need a book. However let me say that the concentration camp reference—like the television presenter's inane statement about men wanting women with curves—only serves to emphasise to the anorexic that they are inadequate, found wanting. What those making the comments do not understand is that the anorexic *does not know how to be what they are told to be*.

There is a gap between what is judged from the outside to be desirable and what the anorexic or bulimic knows they are capable of because, of course, it is the anorexic or bulimic self that hears and feels inadequate and shamed. And this self, now in control, drags the whole person even more deeply into the painful and diseased internal world of the person with an eating disorder. In client-centred terms we are talking about a *self-concept* rather than the *organismic valuing process* (Mearns and Thorne, 1999, pp. 9–10).

Many people with eating disorders develop bizarre (sometimes seen as humorous) manifestations around food. I began to haunt the sweet counters of the big department stores, buying a pound or more of chocolates in their shiny, seductive wrappers and eating them in the privacy of my bedroom. Then I would drink pints of orange juice which I was convinced neutralised the sugar. Then I would refuse dinner saying I was full and spend the evening exercising before finally passing out.

I say 'passing out' because often I did not so much fall asleep as black out. By the time I entered my fully anorexic period—having started at one hundred and fifty pounds I now weighed about one hundred and ten—I was having difficulty finding the energy to get through life. I had left school and at nineteen began working for an advertising agency. The job did not suit me and my unhappiness caused me to focus even more on dieting, exercise and isolation.

Isolation came easily in our family. My parents were unhappily married. They were isolated from themselves and we four children were isolated from each other. Because dysfunction is different for different families, I wonder what other sorts of patterns are prevalent in families with someone with an eating disorder?

I do think that sex plays some sort of role in eating disorders. Not so much the actual act, but the *idea* of being sexual. For myself, knowing (fearing) that I was gay made thinking about sex within our homophobic family even more terrifying. Denial was the only option. Becoming anorexic, therefore, was also a way of putting my burgeoning sexual desires on hold, since by the time my anorexia was at its most powerful I no longer had the energy to produce sperm, so embarrassing night emissions—sleep and dreams had always 'tortured' me with my homosexual secret—completely stopped.

This is also why the television presenter's 'curves' comment is particularly dangerous. Firstly, it presumes the young woman is heterosexual, secondly it humiliates her for not being sexual in the way society demands. I am of the opinion that the reason why eating disorders manifest so often at that point when the adolescent is called upon to assume the mantle of adulthood is that the person feels an obligation to make some sort of jump and does not know how.

By this time, around about twenty, I was swimming every day in an open-air pool throughout the winter. I was so tired by 9.30 a.m that all I wanted to do was go home and go to bed. Yet I was still standing helpfully at the cake trolley, taking slices of chocolate birthday cake or fruit tarts to my fellow workers, careful never to take a single morsel myself.

One morning, I stood on a pair of scales and saw I weighed less than ninety-five pounds. At that moment I had a profound realisation of being seriously ill. But I did not know what to do about it. I had had a couple of incidents in the previous six months when, persuaded by my mother's pleas to eat something nourishing, I had tucked into a cheese fondue and been horrified, at the following morning's weigh-in, to find that I appeared to have gained five pounds overnight. The horror that I could once again become overweight—that I would lose the control I now exercised over food, over myself and my life—manifested itself in a still stricter eating regime with, of course, the infrequent binges, such as devouring two packets of chocolate biscuits on a rare occasion when hunger overwhelmed the controlling anorexic self.

So this was my position. I was unable to put on weight sensibly, able only—under the direction of the powerful anorexic self—to approach each day with more control, more denial, more diseased discipline.

Matters came to a head one weekend when I came home from work on a Friday evening and my mother asked me how the day had gone. I started crying and could not stop. My parents were horrified and said I need not return to the job.

I should explain that, since the anorexic self was in charge, *it* was trying to run my office-life as well. Most nights I spent lying awake worrying desperately about some job that was not where it should be. However, I had another aspect of the disorder that I have noticed in other people with disorders. I had a highly developed, if somewhat 'skewed', sense of responsibility—something that I have since observed in clients who, though unable to look after themselves properly, nevertheless have a noticeable drive towards being responsible for others. Again, in person-centred terms, my self-concept was exhibiting its recognisable characteristics: 'the self-concept is rigid and negative, maintained with the help of powerful defence mechanisms' (Mearns, 1994: 107–8).

Therefore I returned to work on Monday. Once again I broke down and was put on indefinite leave. Now the matter was out in the open. The one medical support I did receive was a course of Vitamin B12 injections. My family, with the exception of my mother, completely ignored my situation. I was left on my own. This is when I experienced for the first time the power innate in each of us to heal ourselves.

I have referred previously to the 'anorexic self'. Years after this period I discovered, in Eastern esoteric philosophy, the idea that we are not one, single, indivisible 'I', but groups of 'I's, some of which are ignorant of others, or even completely antithetical (Ouspensky, 1950, Chapter 2). This makes sense when you think how surprising people can be with their collection of likes and dislikes. And it made a crucial difference to me, struggling on my own.

I knew the anorexic self was powerful. I knew it was merciless. I knew I was seriously ill. And I knew I wanted to live. Not for any specific reason other than I also did not know how to die—so I had no choice but to try to learn how to live. The weak, healthy part of my psyche talked to the stronger, frightened, anorexic part: it negotiated. The deal was not that I would need to eat more in order to recover my health, but that I needed to eat in order to exercise. That was the only way the anorexic self could hear the suggestion.

There is something of the flavour of this idea of different 'I's in Mearns' *Developing Person-Centred Counselling*. He refers to the case of Elizabeth, who named 'competing dimensions' of herself, 'the nun' and 'the little girl' (Mearns, 1994, pp. 12–16). Mearns reinforces my own understanding when he writes:

> A crucial point to note about the work … is that at no stage did the person-centred counsellor push for the separation of these aspects of the personality, nor did the counsellor offer labels to the client for these different parts. (Mearns, 1994: 12–14)

My mother continued to help, buying me exactly what I asked for: fresh fruit, yoghurt, nuts and grains. I still did not usually eat after about 4 p.m., but breakfast and lunch were now fairly respectable meals. One thing I remember—and remember now with a great deal of affection for my wounded but still hopeful body—was the first time I ate a baked potato after two and a half years. The butter, the soft white mashed inside, exploded in my mouth like orgasmic, joyous mini-suns. My poor abused taste buds were taking no chances that I would not understand that *this food was good for me*.

Another specific memory concerned my morning trips to the swimming pool at the nearby University. The journey to the pool was a delightful mile's walk through semi-tropical parkland and going so early allowed me to bypass the man checking student cards. The water was quite cold since, although we were coming into spring, the sun was not up yet. One morning I remember coming to the end of a length, turning over to return and surfacing. My hair was long then and it clung to my eyelids. The sun had just broken free of the horizon and the droplets of water in my eyes caught the first rays. It was an explosion of lights in my eyes. I swam enchanted, laughing with joy, laughing because now I had the energy to laugh.

Recovery, I believe, is built out of random incidents like these. For me, without a map, it was not by following a set order. In fact any attempt to make me follow an order would have resulted in rebellion from the still strong anorexic self. My tentative steps back to a normal eating pattern and a more regular life were delicate: offering rather than pushing the anorexic self. In fact it seems to be that we *cannot* confront our emotions directly because they are not under our control, they have a mind of their own. Therefore I keenly, gently, learned to listen to my senses and rather than impose, I offered.

What has this to do with the person-centred approach? I've gone into this detail to illustrate the depth and sensitivity of the interface that exists between the emotional, intellectual, instinctive and physical bodies. Therefore to impose, externally, any sort of judgement when, internally, there are all these different voices to please is essentially futile.

And Rogers (1959) was aware of this. He wrote that the six conditions are necessary and sufficient for beneficial change. And since I have detailed how so much was going on inside me, how could an outside party have known *better than* me exactly what was going to be acceptable and what not?

I would add (as I have said in this chapter) that part of *counsellor congruence* is making known the other pieces of information that are relevant to this issue and that I have come across. To me, it would be incongruent to have knowledge and not share it with the client: to offer it and have the client take and make of it what sense he or she wants.

Therefore, although there is nothing about the multiple 'I's and the idea of a healthy part liaising with the strong, ill self in client-centred theory, this understanding I made at the time was central to my recovery process.

My mother took a role similar to that of a client-centred therapist. She offered support and practical help. But she did not attempt to push me one way or another. In a way she had tried all the methods she could think of; finally there was nothing left but to let me work it out for myself. This understanding is echoed in the words of Lisa James, a mother whose teenage son, Drew, also developed an eating disorder:

> I found in my experience as a Mum, desperately forcing or trying to get my son to eat, was not helpful—if only it were that simple ... Food was Drew's 'enemy' and he would battle every attempt at my trying to make food his friend again ... I realised we had to look at *why was he doing this and what issues/feelings were underpinning it.* The 'how we could get him to appreciate food and

eat again?' came much later. Firstly Drew needed to reconnect with food by dealing with his feelings. (James, 2006: 4 [emphasis added])

A vital element in my recovery was finding new ways to live. On my wardrobe mirror I began to write notes to myself. 'Eat'. 'Sleep'. 'Rest'. 'Breathe'. 'Enjoy'. On each I carefully included the date. This was because if I had the same thought a week or a month later, but could nevertheless see that I had had the same thought before, it gave me a new sense of continuity: that I could let go of my erratic over-controlling and trust that something healthy, something new and better, was emerging from inside and instinctively knew what was good.

In other words, I was following the path of therapeutic growth. Rogers believed that once the right circumstances were in place, the psyche and body would instinctively make the right choices for a more balanced and healthy way of living. This is the actualising tendency (Rogers, 1951, Proposition VI, pp. 492–4). Here, I realise I had lived his process before I first read about it, when twenty years after my anorexia I began studying for my counselling qualification.

Having battered my body and psyche, not just during the anorexic period but also when I was overweight, I became aware of needing to instil new beliefs. Since becoming a therapist I have sometimes spoken to new clients of my belief in a need to find somewhere inside us where good feelings, good experiences, can 'stick'. This place can then grow inside us, influencing and pervading the old, sick beliefs and fostering a joy and strength inside.

I remember reading about the 'mirror exercise'. You stand in front of a mirror and look deep into your reflected eyes. Apparently when we see something we are attracted to our pupils dilate—we literally 'drink in' the sight. My pupils did not dilate when they looked into my eyes—but it was a thought. If no one else is doing it, look into your own eyes and think, 'I love you'. This I did and was rewarded by a warm internal glow which grew as I continued to do the exercise.

This sort of self-reinforcement is also, I believe, vital in recovery. Particularly in that, if no one else will do it, we can do it for ourselves. Of course, it could be considered an external locus of control to be reliant on anyone else giving us positive reinforcement. The deeper point is that a client is entirely able to do this for him or herself.

Having this sort of healthy independence is the opposite of what is central to anorexia—an unhealthy independence. The anorexic independence is unhealthy because we do have some dependencies—what may be more helpfully thought of as an *interdependence* with life, with food, with others. But the anorexic independence, which begins so proudly with a demonstration of discipline over food and the pleas of others to *eat something*, becomes confused and lost in a psychic quagmire.

In person-centred terms, it's the rising and taking control by the self-concept. I believe the anorexic voice is a clear example of an extreme self-concept. To look back at the beginnings of my own experience in person-centred terms, at the beginning 'I' : what I thought of as my organismic self—trying to lose weight and be attractive to others.

But *not* being in my organismic self—already being principally in my self-concept—

26

when the anorexic voice began to gain influence over the whole I did not recognise what was happening and continued to behave in a way that made the anorexic self stronger.

Another Eastern theory is that these different 'centres' we have—intellectual, emotional, instinctive and the physical body—*fight for each other's energy*. Thus, when we need to make an intellectual decision, our emotions do it; what we might label a 'hot-headed response'. Or we have a difficult meeting ahead—and spend the minutes pacing anxiously (using the physical body) rather than coolly working out our strategy.

In the case of the anorexic self being the self-concept, the anorexic self-concept gains power and energy by taking it from the other centres. Then it is stuck with the task of trying to *manage tasks* which should rightly be managed by the proper 'centres'.

For example, there can be that over-developed and skewed sense of responsibility. An anorexic may starve herself for what would seem to others a fantastical reason; for example, because there are millions starving in other parts of the world. To the anorexic self-concept, it makes sense. A bulimic self-concept might go in for complex relationships—'two-timing' a boyfriend or girlfriend—and then punish themselves with an extended period of physical sickness.

The anorexic self-concept, having been created artificially, cannot draw on the proper resources in the psyche. Panic attacks, paranoia and other manifestations occur because the individual is stuck with the inadequate responses of the self-concept rather than the response being made by the right internal centre.

Therefore, in my process of recovery, what was needed was a return and rediscovery of organismic processing. Little exercises like the mirror one, keeping notes of how I had been before so that I could trust my psyche to be in place and give the right response when needed, caused the balance of power and energy to shift from the self-concept towards the organismic self.

One thing I have emphasised to clients with an eating disorder is that they should not see the self-concept as something hateful or evil. For me in my recovery, part of loving myself was *integrating* the anorexic self-concept into the whole. What I used to say to myself, and what I say to clients, is that the self-concept was doing its best. The fact that it was woefully inadequate is not actually its fault. It is trying to accomplish the task—which is to survive and get the whole person through life.

Of course, what the self-concept finally needs to do is let go, to surrender power, to allow the growing organismic self to instinctively know what is needed. Often clients have reported, in the third or fourth session: 'I do not know what has changed, but I know that something has. Now I have more choice over the decisions I need to make'. Clearly this is the action of the increasingly powerful, organismic process.

Therefore, we are not one, whole 'I'. We have different parts, different motivations, belonging to different physiological parts of us—the intellect, the emotions, the instinctive system and the moving or physical centre. Each of these tries to do the work of others and *steals energy* from other centres.

The self-concept is a rigid, black/white thinker, wildly fluctuating, unable to see beyond a narrow line. Because at the beginning it seems a positive thing, energy grows in an artificial eating disorder. This eating disorder-self has the same characteristics as the self-concept. Additionally, it is desperately frightened and often paranoid and sees no way out other than ritualised behaviour, denial of normal bodily needs and strict discipline.

We cannot fight the eating disorder/self-concept head on—it is rooted in the emotional centre and is not available to our intellectual arguments. It has to be *negotiated with*, it has to be understood for what it is—trying to do a job but with the wrong set of tools.

This is why the correct person to be in charge of the recovery process is the person with the disorder. Only they can make the delicate internal changes, only they can know when they are pushing too hard and can step back to allow the disordered self room to breathe, to calm down.

One precious asset in the recovery process is sleep. When I was in my own recovery I often felt overcome with great waves of tiredness during the day. Because I was not working I was able to take to my bed. When I woke up I felt invigorated, full of new energy and I was aware that something had happened during sleep.

I remembered this when speaking to a client who reported how feeling tired at strange times of the day made her feel irritable. I encouraged her to go with her body's natural rhythm, to sleep when her body asked for it. 'Sleep,' said Macbeth, 'knits up the ravelled sleeve of care' (Act 2, Scene ii). Allowing our body's unconscious and instinctive parts to work while we are asleep, and unable to attempt to meddle, not only accomplishes in sleep what we cannot accomplish with our intelligence but also allows *trust* in ourselves to grow.

Re-finding this trust is another vital part of recovery. If you consider that what has happened in the process of an eating disorder is that the self-concept has taken to itself all sorts of inappropriate bodily functions—breathing, swallowing food and drink—then letting go of those functions, going to sleep and allowing our battered instinctive centre to resume its proper work is clearly not only important but vital to a lasting recovery.

Where is the client-centred counsellor or therapist in this recovery process? A client of mine took several sessions before she acknowledged that she was already seeing another counsellor. This person allowed her to talk about herself, but did not offer any specific understanding of eating disorders. This meant that although the client gained by having someone to talk to, she preferred to come to me where she could be offered information specific to her needs.

Therefore, thinking for yourself about what the process may be and being clear about your role can be the most helpful. I remember another client saying that he had never been able to talk about the extent to which he needed to perform rituals before he was able to eat anything. When he went into details with me I felt momentarily overwhelmed. Into my head popped the thought 'this is too much for me—perhaps he should be in a psychiatric ward'.

The client continued talking while, internally, I searched for a way to be congruent. The idea of a psychiatric ward did not feel like the right solution—how would it help, with what I had experienced, to think that putting power in the hands of doctors would necessarily benefit my client? Then I remembered my own recovery.

What had worked was *negotiation*: internal negotiation between my healthy and anorexic self, quietly, methodically, patiently. This is what I shared with my client and this made sense to him.

Another fear which clients express is 'once I am no longer ill, who will I be?' and 'when I'm no longer talking about my illness, what will I talk about? There seems to be this great black void'.

Here it's appropriate to remind the client about the self-concept, to ask which part of the client has the fear. It is the self-concept talking. The self-concept has no sense of anything outside itself. Not only does it not trust the body to undertake primary functions like breathing and eating *without* its interference, it also cannot see anything beyond itself and the illness other than 'this great black void'.

When a client expressed this, we looked at another aspect of the results of an eating disorder: isolation. In the process of the disorder, attention moves from the external world to the internal. Constant monitoring of bodily functions eats into available energy and becomes all-consuming. Therefore it can appear to the individual that recovery necessitates the appearance of the black void.

What the client needs to hear at this point is that, firstly, it is the self-concept talking—so it needs to be loved, appreciated, thanked—and gently disengaged and allowed to let go. Assure your client that, as their focus begins to move away from the illness and back into the world, the world will move back—perhaps rush in—to fill up the void. Again, it's obviously desirable that recovery take place at the client's pace. I suggested to one client that he go for walks (as long as he felt comfortable with this) in order to give him something other than food to focus on in the morning.

In this way, carefully and at their own speed, the client begins to separate the action of the disorder with other, healthier, uses of their waking hours. A simple daily routine of a walk in the morning, reading of an informative book, writing in a diary, talking to a friend, will begin to instil *balance*. Remember that the centres rob each other—and take advantage of that fact. If a certain amount of energy is being used in non-disorder pastimes, the disorder itself is proportionately weaker and the healthy self can grow.

It is this realignment that was the ultimate secret to my own recovery. There was no dramatic cut-off, blocking or denial of the anorexic self: only that my life took off in other ways and, since my energy was going in other directions, the anorexic self became weaker and was gradually integrated into the whole of me. From my congruence, I told the client who was concerned about the black void that my experience had been that when I really began to embrace the outside world I needed all my energy; I just did not have enough energy to maintain the disorder.

Therefore it's a vital part of the recovery process that what lies beyond the disorder is explored and embraced. For myself, I went to university and took a degree in English and Speech and Drama. As you might imagine, this gave the various parts of me outlet for the angst and grief still emerging from my history. The client concerned about the black void responded enthusiastically to the idea of continuing his education, and began to take classes in his main interest, art, at a local college.

In retrospect, I have thought that I missed out somehow at university by *not* keeping what I had been through somewhere in my consciousness. I was so delirious about being alive I think my ebullience was misunderstood. Had I explained that I felt newly reborn my 'critics' might have understood. So I think it's helpful with a client to encourage them not to turn their back on the past, but to visit it occasionally, appropriately, and to use it as *a source of personal information*.

As I continue to work with clients I remember other facets of my recovery process. But these I have set down were the most helpful. In the thirty years since my illness I have put on some weight, and lost it again. I like to exercise on a daily basis and feel uncomfortable if I go too many days without. Perhaps that is the ancient remnant of anorexia still making a point. Perhaps it's healthier than having no sense of myself physically.

Overall, I can report that I can eat food or not, take exercise in moderation and, basically, it's only when I'm working with a client that I look into their eyes and see back into my own history.

REFERENCES

Campling, M (2006) A DIY cure for anorexia. *Therapy Today, 17*.

James, L (2006) The Drew Strategy. Unpublished notes: personal communication.

Mearns, D (1994) *Developing Person-Centred Counselling*. London: Sage.

Mearns, D and Thorne, B (1999) *Person-Centred Counselling in Action* (2nd edn). London: Sage.

Ouspensky, PD (1950) *In Search of the Miraculous*. London: Routledge and Kegan Paul.

Rogers, CR (1951) *Client-Centered Therapy*. London: Constable.

Rogers, CR (1959) A theory of therapy, personality and interpersonal relationships as developed in the client-centered framework. In S Koch (ed) *Psychology: The Study of a Science, Vol. 3.* (pp. 184–256). New York: McGraw-Hill.

Rogers, CR (1967) A process conception of psychotherapy. In *On Becoming a Person: A therapist's view of psychotherapy* (pp. 125–59). London: Constable.

CHAPTER 4

FROM BOTH SIDES:
THE EXPERIENCE OF THERAPY

GILLIAN PROCTOR AND ANN REGAN

INTRODUCTION

This chapter describes a counselling/therapy relationship from both sides—from the perspective of the client, Ann, and the therapist, Gillian. It describes the changes that Ann experienced as a result of this therapy and is an update on a paper which they wrote jointly (Regan and Proctor, 2001, 2004a, b). The chapter refers to their therapy relationship between 1996 and 1998.

WHO WE ARE

At the commencement of the therapy relationship Ann is a 42-year-old married mother of three, of mixed race ethnicity from a working-class background working as a care worker with people with learning difficulties. Gillian is a 27-year-old white lesbian with no children. She is from a middle-class background and works as a person-centred therapist, employed as a clinical psychologist.

BACKGROUND TO THERAPY: ANN

I came to counselling expecting very little and I've had some experience to support this. I saw my first psychiatrist at thirteen when I was becoming 'difficult'. The fact that my mother was addicted to barbiturates, regularly hospitalised and under the care of one of the psychiatrist's colleagues didn't enter the equation. Her husband, a very disturbed man, who was sectioned on occasions (such was his illness) was under the care of another of this psychiatrist's colleagues. Anyway, he wasn't much good … asked me to draw a few pictures … end of that one.

Inevitably, I came up against the courts. My probation officer at the time said I had a split personality yet I was never referred anywhere. I was only fifteen and felt I should have been offered some guidance—but perhaps I was not quite ready. When I received my first sentence I was seen by a psychiatrist who gave me a preliminary interview. As I was leaving he asked me, 'What makes the world go round?' 'Love,' I replied. He never asked to see me again. Maybe if I had said money, sex, death etc. I would have warranted a second look. End of that one.

Later, when my husband was seeing a psychiatrist, I took the opportunity of asking her advice. It was clear, concise and painful. I didn't listen at the time but some six years later I knew without a doubt she was right. I asked to be referred to her, but it was too late—she'd left the area. My husband got better: I didn't. Still bitter, still angry, I didn't like many people, didn't trust at all.

Over the years I have, at intervals, tried to seek help and my experiences have made me even more cynical. I have recorded past tragedies. One thought stays with me.

About three or four years ago I saw a psychiatrist who clearly needed help himself. He wore a wig for f - - - 's sake! Perhaps that shouldn't matter, but with all his knowledge of self-esteem problems (I imagine he is knowledgeable) he still wore a rug on his head. Anyhow, I visit this guy not knowing what to expect and as I'm talking he butts in … 'I know, I know', he says, 'I've just had a man in here who has worked all his life', etc., etc., 'and he lives in a ground-floor flat. The kids break his windows, the police do nothing.' Oh my God. This is the f - - - - - g doctor! You go in there depressed; you come out f - - - - - g suicidal! It makes me angry that people like this are allowed to practise. We come to you—for whatever reasons, mostly for help—and get *him*. Of course there's no help from a man like that, so what happens if you then just give up? You're back in front of the courts passing your problems on to your children, convinced more than ever that you are beyond help. There are rules, regulations etc. to protect this doctor—and he keeps on 'practising', does no good whatsoever and no-one, it seems, does anything.

INITIAL IMPRESSIONS: ANN

When I went to see Gillian, my expectations were low. I came to my present counselling faded and cynical. I thought Gillian young, well-meaning and ready to tell me what to do: 'Be good, Ann, just be a good girl.' I looked at this young girl and thought 'Oh dear, Pollyanna to the rescue; what on earth are you going to do with an old warhorse like me?' I didn't think she would understand anything about my life. She was very young, not married, and I assumed that her life experiences would be very different to mine. I was sure she wouldn't understand and if she gave me advice, it would be well-meaning but ineffectual. But Gillian didn't tell me what to do as I had expected. I thought she must have the answers because otherwise what's the point? I expected her to say, 'Well, I think this is what you should do'. I expected her to think she knew the answers: to give me advice I didn't need.

As the appointments continued, I was still expecting her to give me some advice, to say what she thought I should do, and I decided that as soon as she did this I'd stop coming to see her. But even when I asked her, she still didn't tell me what to do. Whereas this was frustrating at first, I gradually came to realise it was *my* life and the lack of advice was the main reason I kept coming.

My first impressions were not favourable in terms of her being able to help me—nice, well-meaning, but ineffective I thought. As time progressed I felt respect: the key for me. I do not automatically respect a badge, a name or position, and as my respect for my counsellor increased I did not wish to share my earlier unkind thoughts.

As our counselling relationship developed she began to become a person, rather than just the 'being' in the counselling room. On telephoning for an appointment I was told 'Oh, she's moving house this week', which, for the first time, made me realise that she existed outside that room. Up until then I had come to appointments and talked, or not, as the case may be. I had no responsibility for this other person, nothing was required of me. This was *my* time only. As I began to heal and get better, I could stop being angry and start actually looking at her and wondering about *her* life and accepting that she *had* a life outside the counselling room. This, I remember, was the first thing I knew about Gillian. I had never asked her anything about herself before; it had never occurred to me to do so. By the end of our counselling relationship Gillian had become a real person with a mum and a dad, a cat, a life. This realisation enabled me, I'm sure, to work with Gillian on this paper. I felt as if I was working with an old friend who knew me well, warts and all, and it was OK. I was OK just as I was.

Going back was very revealing for me in terms of self-awareness. I never envisaged such a profound effect. I came to Gillian in the first instance by referral and wanted to please the woman who had referred me by honouring a six appointment contract—which I expected, when completed, would be the end of it. To find myself some years later armed with this self-awareness, and the ability to articulate it still affects me.

INITIAL IMPRESSIONS: GILLIAN

In her first session, Ann talked about the difficulties she had in her marriage. She asked me if I was married and I replied that I wasn't. After this session I felt concerned that she would think my life so different from hers that I wouldn't understand her. I wasn't sure Ann would think that I could understand her life. She talked about not understanding someone whose parents had died and who was still missing them. She felt they were privileged to feel like that. I felt privileged to know that I *would* grieve my parents, privileged to be white and to not encounter racism. There seemed to be a lot of differences in respect of our life experiences; I doubted my right to even attempt to understand Ann—and felt sure that Ann would have similar reservations.

However, I strived to understand her life and her reactions to people. As I heard more about her life and what people had done to her, the reasons why she was so angry with others, and did not trust them, made sense. As I spent more time with Ann, the facts of her life and the differences to mine faded and I related to her feelings about her experiences. I began to feel more comfortable being with her and trying to understand her. Her anger seemed to me to be a perfectly understandable response to how she had been treated and I wondered if this would change, especially considering all the different things and people she had to be angry with. So I was surprised as, over time, our relationship developed and Ann did seem to trust me and to become much less angry and more able to choose when and how to express her anger. I felt very privileged to be trusted by her and to realise that she did seem to feel that I understood something of her life and feelings and how she was. As Ann changed and her anger diminished I was struck and excited by the spontaneity and unselfconsciousness of this change.

Very soon, I began to develop a deep affection for Ann. I enjoyed being with her and looked forward to seeing her. I really liked her sense of humour and felt I could rely on her to be honest about how she felt about what was happening in therapy. I admired her strength and courage to trust me and to believe that something could come out of our relationship despite all the experiences she had had with other people. I felt I could be myself with her as she began to trust me and I felt very comfortable with her.

I was sad when a change of job meant that I could no longer see Ann in therapy. I knew I would miss her and I did continue to think about her and wonder how she was. I also felt sure that she had changed so much and had built up so much confidence in herself and her new way of being that she would be able to continue this change without me.

CHANGE IN THERAPY: GILLIAN

Rogers (1959) elaborates the familiar six conditions necessary and sufficient for constructive personality change in therapy. Ann's description of what helped her change in therapy elaborates clearly her perception of my attitudes of unconditional positive regard (UPR), empathic understanding (EU) and congruence. These attitudes are incorporated into my way of being as a therapist within the principle of non-directivity. Ann agreed that this theory accurately described what was helpful for her.

UNCONDITIONAL POSITIVE REGARD: ANN

I couldn't work it out much myself to begin with but I just gradually began to feel better and calmer. I felt that the therapy was a sort of a lifeline—I didn't really understand how it worked but I didn't think that mattered: getting better was what mattered and understanding it came later. Being listened to and not judged ... the realisation that nobody is born bad ... well *I* wasn't born bad or wicked anyway. She listened, didn't judge, didn't criticise, preach or advise. How I got better beats me—but I did. I went ... she listened ... and I went away. Somewhere along the way I began to lose my hostility to this Pollyanna crap and I started to see things differently. I began to trust—which is something I don't do easily. As I became more comfortable I opened up more and found immense relief at being able to talk without restraint, without shame. I found her non-threatening ... just ready to listen. I wasn't lectured to or talked down to; I wasn't given a label or diagnosis. I felt like an individual. By the end, I didn't feel there was anything that I couldn't tell her.

EMPATHIC UNDERSTANDING: ANN

I didn't want sympathy and Gillian didn't give it. She was just understanding—understanding, not condoning—but understanding maybe about why I got angry or why I got anxious. It seemed to make sense to her or ... if it didn't, she didn't seem confused. I felt quite safe discussing things with her because the worst thing would have been if she didn't understand or couldn't work out where I was coming from. But, even if she didn't, she still didn't judge me—she didn't push me any further than I wanted to go. After coming here for so long I began to trust what she said because I felt that she understood me. I know she understood because of what she said to me ... and she'd say exactly how I felt ... and I felt she knew what I was talking about and it was safe to go on, and she could understand that I still felt things, even when they weren't logical ... and then I didn't feel like I was nuts.

CONGRUENCE: ANN

I have a sceptical and cynical attitude to life and people in general, but now I actually believe some people are genuine and decent and I hope the few I've found stay in my life. You can feel the same way about your counsellors. I know there's an argument for not getting too close and being too reliant etc., but I wonder if you know how difficult it is to actually find someone you can trust? I can only speak from my own experience. This is why good, clever, caring (whatever you want to call the best) counsellors are rare—and you do mourn their loss, because you wonder what turkey you're going to get next. I felt the loss of my counsellor, Gillian, acutely. I felt Gillian spoke to, or rather *listened* to, the child in me and certainly to my bad side—my other self—who I have never really revealed in such depth before. I would rather travel to see a good therapist than visit my local hospital every week to see someone like the tosser I saw before Gillian. His answer was Prozac. I'd like to punch him—a lot!

Throughout various stages of my life I have come across 'professionals' who haven't been very good and have coloured my attitude and added to my cynicism. Now, at last, I realise a lot can be achieved. It is, however, a two-way thing. You need a therapist who has a genuine desire to help you or listen to you, and eventually you begin to feel it—sincerity that is.

NON-DIRECTIVITY: ANN

She was listening, not judging, not asking me to elaborate on things I wasn't ready to elaborate on, not prying. And it was a relief not to be told what to do, because there's only so much you can tell people. If you tell people you're breaking the law you expect them to tell you not to do that ... so you don't tell them. It's quite a relief to say 'this is what I do and it's not a good thing', and for somebody not to pass any comment at all.

Then I stopped expecting and began to respect her.

PROCESS OF CHANGE: GILLIAN

Rogers (1959, 1961) describes the common processes of change that clients go through in person-centred therapy. He describes how in reciprocity with the therapist attitudes, the client increases in their positive self-regard, self-understanding and congruence. He also describes how as clients change, they are likely to become more aware of their own inner experiencing and to more accurately experience perceptions, become increasingly open to experience and increase in existential living. Ann agreed that all these characteristic processes were true of her.

PROCESS OF CHANGE: ANN

Once you feel safe, and able to trust the person you're talking to, the benefits flow and you feel them for a long time afterwards. It takes a while to build up the trust and you feel at first it will never come. Whether or not you like the person at first is immaterial—you just unload. Then you begin to feel vulnerable: a very uncomfortable feeling. But at some point it's OK to say what you feel and not worry. We're all the same, us hard bastards, we despise weakness. Forgiveness is stupidity—and trust—never! When you shake off the armour, the burden of always being strong, tough, you see so much more clearly and become smarter, more intelligent.

I felt a change in myself, an understanding of myself that still continues. I also feel grateful—a gratitude that will last as long as I do. Grateful for the release of the tension I felt and that I felt understood. So all my initial expectations came to nothing. I had only to give myself a chance, and my prediction that it would all come to nothing didn't happen. I was wrong and happy to be so.

When I see Gillian now, it's like seeing an old friend that I feel comfortable with—more comfortable perhaps because this 'old friend' knows things I've never told anyone; things that she heard without judgement, criticism, pity or advice—that she just listened to. I feel I could say anything to her—just that—say anything without any expectation other than that she would listen to me. It's a relief to have that in your life.

UNCONDITIONAL POSITIVE SELF-REGARD: ANN

I started to think about things differently and see things from where I am now rather than where I was as a child, and now I think maybe I'm not as bad as I thought I was—maybe I'm not nuts; so what's the other possibility? Maybe it's that people become damaged and perhaps if, in my case, I'd been brought up in a different family I'd have been a totally different person. That's something that never occurred to me before my sessions with Gillian. Now I try to be *aware* with my children and to not do what was done to me because I don't want them to be like me. I can make that association for others but, until now, I couldn't do it for myself. It's been quite a revelation.

SELF-UNDERSTANDING: ANN

The way I was treated was appalling—and the more I say that the better I feel. I didn't used to make the connection at all but that's what talking about it has done. I'd talk about it and go away and think, 'That wasn't a nice thing to do to a little girl! Maybe that's why I'm like that'. I've made connections between what I feel like now and what happened to me, and that has only happened by talking about it.

RESULT OF CHANGE IN THERAPY: ANN

I have changed in so many ways; some of them dramatic, some subtle. I am no longer predictable to others. I can feel myself getting angry and can interrupt myself, slow down, change tack or walk away—impossible before, getting easier now. Before, it was like getting on a roller coaster and having to finish the ride. Now I can choose not to get on. I began to realise so much. I accepted that I was very anxious—a statement which at one time I would have deemed preposterous. I always thought myself strong (which I am in some ways) but always there was this anxiety. I'm fully aware of this now and I have my own coping strategies to deal with it. It has been a journey of self-discovery, cliché though that may sound. I thought I was a wicked person with an ungovernable temper and that I was out of control and simply could not be helped. I could not help myself so how could anyone else help me? I knew I was two different people (at least)—well let's say I suspected it. I knew that what I did when I was angry afforded me no remorse, only when I came back down to earth was I sorry—sometimes.

I have a recollection of an incident not very remarkable, but it sticks with me. About eleven or twelve years ago my life was in a constant state of high tension. My marriage was violent and I was always irate. I left home to go into town to do whatever, came home, made tea etc. Tidying up, I discovered a bank receipt detailing a withdrawal from my account. I wasn't too happy. Next day I went back into town and into the bank and as I approached the cashier I had a vague sense of déja vu; it was me who had withdrawn the money the previous day and I had no recollection of it whatsoever. It was only as I approached the cashier, who was in the same place wearing the same clothes, that the memory was revived. That was so frightening as these episodes had happened to me a lot. When I used to be in an angry state it was extremely difficult for me to remember, in my calmer moments, what I had done. I rarely have that problem now and then not to such a degree. Counselling this time around has been, and still is, an enriching part of my life. I now know and believe that I was damaged in the early part of my life and I can see quite clearly where my anxiety comes from—and knowing this makes things easier. I can point out to myself that my anxiety is unreasonable and this is the reason why: I have learned through listening to myself talk and going away and thinking about what I've said, that the life I had as a young girl was wholly unacceptable, and that now, forty years on, I would have (I hope) been treated differently. I can now see quite clearly the cruelty and the neglect, and how it has all affected me. I was angry because I didn't know what else to be. My anger was real and very intense and I could not control it. I avoided situations that I felt would incite me but now I feel able to reach the challenges: stronger and more able.

I have buried so many things and on occasions I've spoken about them for the first time, and it really seems to help. I don't know how; you can't go back and change anything, but you can understand yourself a bit better. All this has led to a better understanding of my life and I am much more complete as a person. I know that now, more than ever, I am not fragmented. I came to look forward to my meetings. I knew I was different, I know that I can't go back (nor do I want to) to how I was. I'm happy that I gave myself the chance to heal. It is an ongoing process and there is still much to do. However, after the time that's passed and the changes I feel and see, and that others see in me, I know I did the right thing.

I noticed a dramatic change in myself about a year into counselling. A woman I particularly dislike was sitting on a bench as the car I was in drew to a stop (I was taking a client shopping). Usually, the sight of this woman would set off a chain reaction in me and I would have gone on to make a scene (I once had to leave Tesco's mid-shop as I didn't trust myself to be in the same shop). Well, I got out of the car, helped my client and walked past her. Nothing. By the time I'd got halfway around the shop the incident had passed from my mind. When I thought about it later, I realised I didn't feel that stomach churning rush that set my heart racing and propelled me towards the inevitable.

When I next saw Gillian I complained. 'What's happened to me? Where's the old Ann gone?' You would think I'd be grateful. That's what I'd always wanted—to be free of that anger—but I felt vulnerable and was grumpy about the loss of my friend. What if this lack of feeling happened when I was in need? What then? Where's she gone? As I got used to the idea I was amazed that I could 'behave' with no effort, and it was a feeling of freedom. This was a chance happening. I'd no time to prepare for it and I was empowered much more than if I'd lost control and made things harder for myself.

I think with my start in life I haven't done too badly, and now with this insight into myself I can do so much better and think things through (unheard of before), and I sleep so much better too. I expect in a year or so I will have changed some more, and so it goes on. I didn't think I'd ever really talk about the things I've done and what's happened to me, but this has been the most important transformation in my life—and I could have done with it long ago.

CONCLUSION

Ann's description of therapy is a clear illustration of how the core conditions were experienced by her as a client. It is also a clear example of the effectiveness of these core conditions for personality change. Ann describes changes that fit well with Rogers' theory of the process of change; she describes changes which go beyond the idea of 'symptom relief' and seem to be better described by the concept of personal development, a process which continues well beyond the end of therapy. This story is also an illustration of the power of person-centred therapy, particularly with problems that could easily be medicalised; demonstrating the power of understanding and accepting rather than diagnosing and medicating.

We met again to write this chapter and Ann was pleased to be able to make sense of her experiences of change using person-centred theory. (She was already aware of some of this having done a counselling course herself since therapy to try and make sense of what had happened.) It was useful and reassuring for Gillian, similarly, to be able to map Ann's experiences of change with what she was aiming to do as a therapist and reaffirm her faith in person-centred theory.

REFERENCES

Regan, A and Proctor, G (2001) Completing the jigsaw: An experience of therapy. *The Journal of Critical Psychology, Counselling and Psychotherapy, 1*, 242–51.

Regan, A and Proctor, G (2004a) Ann's story: An experience of therapy. Part 1. *Healthcare Counselling and Psychotherapy Journal, 4*, 14–18.

Regan, A and Proctor, G (2004b) Ann's story: an experience of therapy. Part 2. *Healthcare Counselling and Psychotherapy Journal, 4*, 22–5.

Rogers, CR (1959) A theory of therapy, personality and interpersonal relationships as developed in the client-centered framework. In S Koch (ed) *Psychology: A Study of Science: Vol. 3, Formulations of the person and the social context* (pp. 184–256). New York: McGraw-Hill.

Rogers, CR (1961) *On Becoming a Person: A therapist's view of psychotherapy.* Boston: Houghton Mifflin.

CHAPTER 5

SURVIVING SOCIAL DISADVANTAGE: A TESTIMONY TO COURAGE

TRACEY SANDERS AND JUNE O'BRIEN

AN INTRODUCTION

Writing a case study is an impossible task. How, when every single interaction between two human beings is so full of experiencing and meaning, can one possibly summarise two years of intense therapeutic work in a few thousand words? Is it, in any case, possible to write such a study without in some way reducing the person concerned to an object who exists to validate the work of the therapist of the therapeutic approach? How tempting might it be to embellish a little and paint the whole therapeutic encounter with an unrealistic gloss?

And yet I feel I must try. For the sake of ourselves, our clients and the work that we do together, we must be willing to examine, communicate and reflect upon what happens in therapy. What seems important to me, then, is that I approach this task in a way which is realistic and which makes clear my intentions and motivations in so doing.

Since I first trained as a counsellor I have felt drawn to working with people who are disadvantaged in our society. I have been lucky to meet many remarkable people whose courage and integrity have affected me deeply. June, the client in this case study, is one of these people. She has participated without disguising her identity and offers some of her own thoughts about the value of counselling and her ongoing journey later on in the chapter. I chose to write about the work June and I did together for many reasons—some practical and some philosophical. I have come to the conclusion that one of my primary motivations is the desire to bear witness to the courage and integrity she—and many others like her—show in living with, and growing through, severe abuse and deprivation. Interestingly, in a recent phone call about this work June, unprompted, used the same words. She had, she said, needed someone to bear witness to her suffering.

At times I have become only too painfully aware that, even in the counselling and psychotherapy world, people are unable to look beneath the surface and to see the qualities present in people who may not conform to stereotypes of acceptability—to see the depth of understanding that is present even when it is not expressed in a nice, neat, 'middle class' sort of way. Counselling and psychotherapy, as a profession, remains chronically middle class in the majority of its values. This is an aspect of our practice which I believe needs serious examination, especially if we wish to promote social justice and personhood rather than colluding with dehumanising and discriminatory forces in our society. Our society tends to value intellect above integrity, wealth creation above personal courage, status above simple humanity. My passion is for a practice of counselling and psychotherapy which, in its very being, challenges the prevailing discourse and meets each person in humility and openness.

Like so many people in her position, there is no way that June could have afforded to pay for private counselling. Fortunately, she was able to access the service I offered for free at a women's project. Our initial eight-week contract became indefinite (thanks to a change in my circumstances) and, in the end, we worked together for two years on a weekly basis. Our work was not finished. We could and would have carried on working together had my personal circumstances not made me unable to continue at that time.

Counselling for more than a few weeks is not available for most people, even when their difficulties are severe and they would benefit from longer-term help. Help, if it is available at all, is only provided to those who are willing to allow themselves to be processed through the machinery of the mental health system—acquiring diagnoses and submitting to 'treatment'. Such help is, most often, qualitatively different from the therapeutic space which I set out to offer. I think it is unlikely that June would have accessed a service which demanded assessment and diagnosis. She was a hesitant client living in a disadvantaged area. Many people in this position have had experience of 'authorities' which is negative and invalidating. They will, understandably, do all they can to avoid situations in which they make themselves subject to relationships in which they fear they will be judged, disempowered and discredited. Without access to help which is humanising, relational, and largely unconditional, offered within an approachable, non-statutory setting, people like June are left to do the best they can to cope alone, sometimes with tragic consequences. It is ironic that any help that is available is generally offered through charities with minimal resources and relying mostly upon unpaid, inexperienced counsellors, despite the very complex needs of their clients.

In any attempt to examine and evaluate our own work it is crucial that clients play a key role. We therapists have too much to gain from presenting our work in a positive light and too much to lose from examining closely its limitations, especially as such limitations will often reflect our personalities and our personal difficulties in relating. One rarely reads case studies about therapeutic failures, or even accounts of feelings of inadequacy and mistakes. This can mean that written accounts of therapy provide a slightly unreal impression of a process that proceeds always to a clear, positive outcome.

In real life, in my experience, this is often not the case. Interruptions occur, relationships split, clients leave without a clean ending, and people go so far and then need time before they are ready to carry on again. All too often we do not really know the outcome of our endeavours, even though we may be confident that the client has benefited from the time they have had and whatever it is we have been able to offer.

This case occurred several years ago. June and I have written with the benefit of a longer-term view of what we did together but without the benefit of notes, tapes or fresh memories. What we can both offer is some of our personal, subjective recollections and meditations upon the particular counselling relationship we shared. First I will

41

share my reflections and what I learned from our time together. Later in the chapter June will write about her experience for herself. I will then respond and close the chapter.

TRACEY'S EXPERIENCE

I have been surprised by how many hesitations I have had to engage with before feeling able to write this chapter. Aside from the philosophical issues referred to earlier there is the immense responsibility of being true to my client. I was unprepared for how conscious this would make me of every word that I write, not to mention the issue of how June might feel reading it. I want to write in a truthful and unreserved way about my experience of the relationship but to do this will involve exposing parts of myself that June has not previously seen and which I may, in any case, be rather shy of sharing with the world. Yet not to do so would, I feel, be to engage in a subtle dishonesty which perpetuates the myth that, in life, some of us are OK and others are not.

There is room for my insecurities too. I am not sure I know what I meant to this client, nor what her long-term assessment of the benefit of our work together might be. I certainly did not choose this case because I regarded it as my most successful or dramatic work. Doing this case study means confronting some of my fears about my own value and the value of the work we did together, and finding out from her, several years on, whether there has been any lasting benefit.

In writing about my experience of working with June I realise that I may leave you with a stronger sense of June's impact upon me than of my impact upon her. I do not apologise for this. Firstly, I would argue that our own experience is ultimately all any of us can speak about; we cannot speak for another. Furthermore, as a therapist committed to a person-centred phenomenological approach I find myself agreeing with Larner (1999: 47) when he says, 'It is not the client's story that is deconstructed so much as the therapist's'.

I venture that it is the very act of allowing the meeting with the client to deconstruct our own stories which enables the client to locate their own power and start to reconstruct the narrative of their own life, whether or not either client or therapist are aware that is what is happening at the time. It is only in such an encounter that our clients experience themselves being met as persons.

Fundamentally, this is about issues of power. It is about a way of relating to others which does not objectify, diminish or categorise them; which does not presume to 'know' who they are or what they need; which does not patronise, does not judge but rather meets them as an equal within the mysterious process of living and is open to learning from them as well as giving to them. This is a responsive and unique interaction in which the counsellor will need all of their humanity and personhood as well as all the courage, understanding and knowledge they can muster in the service of the client. This, it seems to me, is particularly important in working with people who have repeatedly experienced themselves as powerless and abused in relationship with others, especially when this is combined with deprivation and disadvantage. It is, I hypothesise, in this process of experiencing their own power in relationship to another that much subtle but significant change is able to occur.

When I first met June she was at a crucial moment in her life. She and her sister had just taken their brother to court for the sexual abuse they had both suffered at his hands during their childhood. He had been found guilty but was awaiting sentence. Their family had sided with him and the whole thing had been an enormous ordeal. June had hoped that, having achieved a guilty verdict, she would find herself free of the awful burden of those experiences and be able to move on with her life. Unfortunately it was not so simple. June found herself beset by the trauma and emotion of it all and, far from being free, felt very much in the grip of her past.

I never thought about June in terms of a diagnosis but I am sure there are many others that would and could have applied to her at the time. Her life was extremely difficult, punctuated by violence and instability. She and her husband were out of work and living on benefits in an inner city area, doing the best they could to raise three children in really trying circumstances. June was tormented by intense anxiety, outbursts of uncontrollable rage and terrible flashbacks. These made her both intensely vulnerable and emotionally volatile.

I immediately liked and warmed to June. Her energy and honesty were clear to see and easy for me to like. Perhaps more significantly, I was filled with respect for what she had already achieved. I had worked with enough survivors of sexual abuse to understand the enormity of what she and her sister had done. Despite the odds being stacked against them, despite the twenty years that had passed, despite the disbelief of their family and despite the emotional cost involved they had taken the huge step of going to the authorities, reporting their abuse and giving evidence at their brother's trial. That takes enormous courage and is done at significant risk. To look so closely into the past, to make it public and to risk the disbelief of others takes incredible courage, especially when those who have been abused are so often vulnerable to feelings of self-blame and a profound lack of self-worth.

In reflecting now upon my journey with June over the following two years I believe that this respect for what she had done probably played a significant part in making it relatively easy for me to trust her even at times when her difficulties were severe and danger seemed all too close. A profound belief in the right and ability of each person to determine their own way forward underpins both my own personal philosophy of life and my commitment to working in a person-centred way. However holding such confidence is not always easy when faced with a client in considerable distress who has no faith in their own worth and is tortured by the past. Looking back I realise that with some clients I have struggled considerably more to believe in them at those times when they were facing severe and enduring difficulty.

The sessions themselves were, I would suggest, largely unremarkable and characterised predominantly by careful empathic tracking. I find it quite hard to, with confidence, stand back and have a sense of how my presence was experienced by June. Certainly I remember very few 'eureka moments', only an ongoing and deepening exploration of her life and her inner world. We quickly and relatively smoothly developed a trust in each other and June would each week pour out whatever was foremost for her. We laughed, cried, grieved, raged and worried together in all the ups and downs and sideways moments of her life. Some weeks this would be almost mundane and others weeks it would be full of intense, overwhelming emotion.

In the course of two years we must have, at some point, explored almost every aspect of June's life. June was a deeply sensitive, caring and spiritual person who seemed to me to have far more intelligence than her circumstances had allowed her to develop. She had that special knowledge and spiritual sense which is so often, in my experience, present in those who have suffered. She was profoundly aware of the feelings and suffering of others, even those who had caused her great pain. She could see that the pain that they inflicted had been a product of the pain inflicted upon them and showed great compassion towards them, at considerable cost to herself. She also looked back and recognised how she herself had inflicted pain on others through her own distress, deeply regretting the bullying she perpetrated at school and her ongoing struggle with her own rage.

She searched within and outside of herself for some sense of peace and began, in small ways and in fleeting moments, to find some. She began to recognise the ways in which her anxiety caused her to feel responsible for the protection of others and then to experience intense frustration when she could not control what they were doing. A stronger sense of herself began to emerge, including the realisation that her own needs were legitimate and that it was OK for her to try to meet them—a sense of the life that she wanted to have and a growing sense that it might be possible. Change was gradual and mostly occurred whilst we weren't looking—the trademark, for me, of organic change which was arising unforced from subtle yet significant changes in June's self-concept and self-experience.

As we moved along, events emerged that gradually took her forward. She went on a trip to Australia. This was a huge step and an achievement to leave her family behind and go exploring for a month. She completed a course in massage, for which she had a natural talent, and in doing so faced many of her own fears about studying. One day she got a job, not cleaning but caring, and she has continued in a variety of roles up to the present. She started taking less responsibility for others and more for herself. She became more available to her children and husband and less consumed by fear. These changes may seem easy and quick written here but of course they were not. Each of them represented a challenge in itself and brought many hurdles to be overcome.

Violence was and always had been a big part of June's experience in a way which those of us who have led more sheltered lives may find hard to imagine. Her childhood was filled with violence, both physical and sexual, and mostly perpetrated by men on women. She lived in a society where violence was commonplace and nothing about her world felt safe or easy or comfortable. On those many occasions when she would explore her childhood and relive the emotions associated with it there was, for me, an extraordinary bleakness about it. It was quite simply filled with fear, violence and poverty. Sometimes I would go home and weep at the sheer awfulness of what she had shared with me. I am aware that some might see this as a sign of inappropriate over-involvement. I feel, however, that to have been with June on her journey without allowing myself to be affected by it would have been to have let go of my humanity in the service of supposed professionalism. I was not overwhelmed, nor engulfed, nor unable to remain secure in my sense of myself and my own life. On the contrary it was important for me to allow myself the time and space to process the emotional impact of what I was hearing in a way which enabled me to carry on being open to June at a subtle and emotional level. I was appropriately distressed by the suffering of another human being with whom I was in relationship.

It is not easy to stay with such distress and I believe I was altered by the experience. In order to remain open to June's pain I had to open further to my own. It is hard to describe in words, but to receive such distress requires a willingness to meet the other in all their suffering without seeking to alter, defend against or even alleviate it. The openness of which I am speaking has, for me, something of the quality which I believe Carl Rogers indicates in his definition of positive regard, 'To perceive oneself as receiving positive regard is to experience oneself as making a positive difference in the experiential field of another' (Rogers, 1959: 208).

This captures for me the sense of positive regard as an experiential openness to and embracing of the other in all their aspects, the sense that the other person's impact is not feared or pushed away or even tolerated, but that the whole of the other is welcomed into one's experiential field. It is, by definition, without judgement, agenda or malice. The term 'positive' implies a duality with which I am not comfortable however, especially as it is too easily confused with approval. I like John Welwood's use of the term 'unconditional presence' (Welwood, 2000: 147) and believe this, for me, more accurately sums up the heart of what I believe Rogers was pointing to in the notion of unconditional positive regard. Unconditional presence is what I hope I was fairly consistently able to offer to June during our time together.

I believe this has spiritual connotations. We cannot maintain a belief in 'happy endings' or 'happy families' if we allow ourselves to open to such suffering. We cannot think that the world is safe, or just, or fair. We cannot feel ourselves to be exempt from the possibility of tragedy .We cannot pretend that people 'only get what they deserve'. When we come to experience the suffering of another on an existential level we see that they are just like us, and all our defences against the awful possibilities of life are shattered. The risk of living is laid bare.

I want to be clear here that, in saying all of this, I by no means wish to negate all that is beautiful, marvellous and awe-inspiring in life. I have a strong spiritual sense and am strongly drawn to a mystical view of life. I hold within my heart the possibility that everything in our existence is a manifestation of love, and at times in my life I have sensed this so clearly that I could almost touch it.

At other times more malign possibilities have seemed much more real. It is possible that everything is meaningless; it is possible there is no higher power or spiritual force; it is possible there is no meaning or solace in suffering; it is possible that our existence has no purpose beyond itself.

I do not know what is true, nor can I hope to do so, and what is true for me may not be true in the life of another. I may have known moments of solace, comfort, ecstasy and joy—others may have had quite a different experience. If I need their view and experience of life to accord with, and perhaps validate, mine then I cannot be open to how life is for them. If I am open to how life is for them then I have to open myself to the uncertainty of my own view of reality.

With June, and in other things which were happening in my life at the time, I learned to be more open to a certain level of suffering in which the soul is tortured. Strangely, one of the manifestations of this was in my use of the word 'fuck'. It was a word I had always chosen consciously not to use. I found it an ugly word, violent even, especially with its sexual connotations. It was not a word I ever wanted to use. June used it all the time. It was quite a crucial part of her vocabulary and that of many people around her. Of course I was quite used to other people using it and was not at all bothered by this. Somewhere along the line, however, I began, in accompanying June, to perceive the word differently. Its sexual meaning was lost altogether and replaced instead with the sense of being profoundly stuck, frustrated, trapped, tormented (all the terms that come most readily to mind in describing this are also swear words). I heard how, for June, it expressed her suffering in a way that other words would not do. And I began to use it myself to describe my pain and that of others. I now use it quite frequently, rather casually at times, but mostly to convey a certain sort of psychic pain—a sore and painful place.

I guess, from all of this, that the reader might gather that at times June and I were exploring dark territories. I could be with June and still maintain a sense of my own inner stability most of the time. On other occasions June's material would trigger my own fears and I would find it much more difficult not to be drawn into a place of anxiety in myself. When that happened my fear would become difficult to contain and I very much needed the support of supervision in order to maintain my own balance. I was fortunate in having a supervisor who understood and valued what we were doing and was able to be the rock I needed to steady myself when it all got a little too close.

The danger and violence that had been in the past was still all too apparent in the present. I often think that people who live deprived lives suffer more trauma in a year than many of us suffer in a lifetime and that was certainly true for June. Everyone around her was suffering in their own way and trauma, insecurity, illness and violence were commonplace. Explosive situations would arise and no-one could possibly predict their outcome. Sometimes the line between near-miss and tragedy was only wafer-thin.

Most distressing of all, June herself, in moments of great anxiety, distress and frustration, would lose control and lash out at those around her—often those that she loved the most. She was terrified of what might happen and filled with remorse, yet she was also powerless to prevent herself exploding when she was pushed beyond endurance. This was, I believe, one of the areas in which most change occurred during our time together.

When we first started working together the rages would arise without warning and felt totally outside June's control. Gradually however, perhaps largely as a result of the changes to June's sense of self that I discussed earlier, June started to gain insight into how these times arose. She became more aware of the stresses that built up and how these might be triggered into an overwhelming rage. She began to be able to monitor in

46

herself the gradual build up that occurred and to start to find ways of dealing with the issues differently.

One incident always sticks in my mind and may have been something of a turning point. This particular week the whole situation around June seemed full of danger. Violence was being threatened by several people involved in a bitter dispute and anything could have happened. It would only have taken a tiny spark for serious violence to erupt—the sort of small coincidences which invariably contribute to tragedy and which no-one could possibly control. There was a real possibility that someone would get seriously hurt, and it might be June who would do the damage.

I cannot say now whether the danger that week was greater than at other times. What I do know, however, was that we were both acutely aware of the danger of the situation. We could see it coming.

We spent a very emotional hour with June expressing her anger, frustration, fear and helplessness. I did nothing except seek to stay with her in it as best I could and to express my understanding of what she was feeling. After she left, acute anxiety descended upon me. What if something awful were to happen? Was there more I could or should have done? At the time it had felt entirely right to just *be* with her in all she was experiencing but how would I feel if something awful were to happen? Was empathy, companionship, presence enough or did I have a responsibility to *do* something? What, in any case, could I possibly have done?

It was one of those, thankfully rare, occasions when the emotional impact of the session stayed with me throughout the week. I went along to the following session full of nervous anticipation. I was relieved when she appeared and seemed to be OK. She started telling me about her week and began describing a situation where her husband had been angry with her and had been verbally provoking her. She could sense what was happening inside her and knew that if he kept on she would 'blow': she would reach the point where she could no longer stop herself reacting and attack him physically. If she was able to reach him then there would be no telling what she might do. She described how she went upstairs and into their bedroom, with him following her, continuing his provocation. The tension was palpable as I wondered what had happened next.

My nerves were at a peak when June described how she had picked up a hammer. What she had done with it was a surprise that I never could have foreseen. Knowing how close she was to exploding into violence, and wanting to protect everyone from the consequences of that, June had used the hammer to nail the bedroom door shut from the inside. In that way, even if she could no longer control herself she knew she would be unable to reach her husband and could do him no harm.

I was flabbergasted and relieved. Then, and now, I remain humbled by the courage, self-awareness and determination June showed in those moments. It is a powerful testament to the strength of the human spirit. It was an act of profound self-control, at a level that I believe most of us can only imagine. I also wonder whether it was significant therapeutically. In those moments June proved to herself that, even when events were pushing her beyond breaking point, she was able to find a way to prevent herself from hurting others. She was able to find her own power even in a moment of intense powerlessness. Certainly it seemed to spark within her a greater sense of her need and, most significantly, ability to change her relationship with her anger, as she had also been to the library and taken out a book on anger management.

It will have become apparent that I was very fond of June and enjoyed her presence. The superficial differences between me and June are obvious for anyone to see—accent, education, class, manner, vocabulary and dress. But in our counselling room I was far more aware of the similarities. I am the same age as June and throughout our work together I know I was affected by a profound sense that all that separated us, in truth, was the accident of birth. I am not sure that I would have coped as well with all that she has had to endure.

Confronted with the depth of courage and integrity which June brought to our sessions, I found myself feeling, once again, that the awareness she displayed (like that of others like her) was greater than that of many who claim to be aware. And her achievements in life were more meaningful than those of many who are lauded in our society.

JUNE'S EXPERIENCE

When I met Tracey I thought I didn't need a counsellor but I went along because one of the women at the project encouraged me to do so. I thought because I had confronted my brother in the court case all the pain, anger and hurt would go away. Little did I know that all those feelings were going to be unleashed and I would have to look at them full on in order to stop them destroying me.

I was always a talker and I felt I could talk to anyone, make them laugh and try to get them to like me. So that is how it started with Tracey—I would talk, crack jokes, talk about my kids and husband, anything to avoid the real hurt inside me. But she kept coming back week after week until I started to trust her. I really wanted to talk but I had to know she would listen. Listening was what she did for two whole years—she listened and listened about the court case against my abuser, my shitty life, my family, my own sins and wrong doing, she listened to it all.

I don't think Tracey ever knew just how much those sessions saved me from committing suicide. Sometimes I would go home after them and scream and smash things in the house because of the feelings which were churning within me. I was too frightened to tell Tracey at the time because I was afraid she would judge me or think I was mad. At other times my emotions would cripple me and I would not get out of bed. I would spend the time in between sessions trying to understand how I felt, trying to feel the rage, without the violence, to feel the pain without wanting to hurt someone in return.

Talking my feelings through with Tracey helped me to realise that these feelings are mine and to learn to live with them. At the sessions I could get angry, lose control and even cry. That was a big thing for me—to be able to cry in front of people and still be in control. It was possible because I knew that Tracey was willing to be there with all my feelings and not judge me for my own wrong doing (including the bullying I inflicted on others and the hurt I have caused other people). I don't want to be full of hate and anger, I want to live my life to the full and be happy, especially for me, my husband Pat and my kids. I cannot change what has already been done and I know I still have this violence raging within me but because of those counselling sessions I can live a life as close to normal as possible.

Counselling allowed me to be as honest as I could be at the time. I don't know if I ever got to the real depths of all my feelings or was a hundred per cent ready to look at myself that deeply but I do know that talking helped me immensely. It allowed me to find new ways of expressing myself, even my anger found a way to vent itself. I still carry all my feelings now, albeit at a lesser intensity. Even today, I can still have what others call my 'mad moments' where I scream and rant but the difference is that I don't throw plates anymore and I rarely smash things. Instead I handle my anger by walking my dogs until I calm down enough to find the words to tell my husband Pat what is on my mind. He is one of the few people I trust in the world and he loves and understands me.

When I was a child, before I ever met or knew what a counsellor was, I didn't have anyone to talk or turn to when I was being raped and abused. Nothing will ever change that fact. Even as a kid I knew that when the sexual abuse ended (and I knew it would end one day) it would never go away for me. I knew I would live with the memories, the filthy words whispered in my ear, the loneliness in thinking I was the only one this was happening to, the brainwashing that made me believe that no-one would believe or listen to me should I ever find the words.

As a child I didn't have the words to express the anguish that I felt on the inside, I had no words to tell anyone what was happening to me or to explain what was going on in my mind. Even now I have big problems expressing myself. I find it very difficult to state the fact that I was raped—I use the term 'abuse'. Only a few people know all the details of the abuse and my sister, nephew and friends are the only people I can call family. I cherish them all.

I always knew deep inside I would survive, albeit inside I felt and still do feel broken. Life throws things at you and you determine how you handle it and what it is going to do to you. I tried the alcohol, I tried the drugs, I tried all sorts of things to get rid of the feelings, to put them in a different place, to make them easier to cope with but there is no other place—it is always there and it never goes away.

Now I am older I don't want the feelings to go away. They are a big part of me—not the most important bit but important none the less—part of who I am and who I am becoming. Because of all my experiences I am learning to accept all of myself, feelings and all. Deep inside I always knew I would survive. I always had a determination to live a good and happy life and I believe I am succeeding.

I still cry for my mother and the rest of my family but not to the point that my grief can destroy me. I still have my mad days where I rant and scream but I am blessed with a wonderful partner and children who are able to laugh at me and have taught me to laugh at myself. I have survived thanks to Pat my husband who has stood by me through all my moments of madness. I never really believed he loved me but now I know he loves me and, even more importantly, I can allow myself to be loved by him and my wonderful children whom I treasure above all other people.

Today I am forty-one years old and surviving. I am blessed in many ways. I am growing, changing and looking forward to my future. I believe in God and I raged at Him when I was younger. Now I know terrible things happen every day in the world and everyone suffers some trauma which can define them if they allow it to. Knowing that does not help me to accept what is happening: that children are still being hurt and abused every second of every day. I feel overwhelming sadness and anger whenever I hear of a child who has been abused. Nevertheless I choose not to allow the abuse I endured to define who I am. I choose the path that I walk.

REFLECTIONS AND CONCLUSIONS

June's powerful words convey both the trauma of the experiences she has lived through and her ongoing courage in seeking to live a life which is not defined by her abuse. They also highlight that, for her, time was an essential component of the trust that developed between us within the counselling relationship and that this deepening of trust was an ongoing process. If June and I had met for only eight weeks we might have done some valuable and worthwhile work but, as June indicates, we would not have got beyond a largely superficial level of relating. June needed to be sure that I would listen and accept her before she could begin to relate to me at depth and start to reveal the full extent of her despair and suffering—trust needs to be earned rather than being offered without question, and time is essential if this is to happen. I should not be surprised by this for it mirrors my own experience as a client, counsellor and trainer. I believe this is true for most clients and is especially important for people whose trust has been repeatedly betrayed and abused. This natural and valuable self-protective mechanism needs to be respected if people are to be allowed to look after themselves. This has major implications at a time when short-term therapy is generally the only option available to people who cannot afford to pay for their own counselling. There is a danger that many people who have much to gain from a stable, long-term therapeutic relationship will be the least likely to gain access to such help.

Furthermore, even after two years, that process of deepening trust was not complete. It would have deepened further had we had more time. Talking to June now I am touched by her sense of loss about the work we were not able to do because our counselling relationship came to an end. In particular she is aware that she would have been able to have looked more deeply into her feelings towards her mother and perhaps seen a way forward with this relationship. This is certainly an area which I remember being a theme in our final months together. Much though June values the support she receives from her family and friends, she has missed a space where she could carry on the process of exploration which takes place within a person-centred relationship. As she said to me, she doesn't want other people's solutions—they don't fit her values; what she wants is the space and the understanding which will enable her to find the solutions that feel right for her. Whilst she gained much from our time together that has enabled her to live more fully she is aware that allowing herself to continue to unfold her strong and painful feelings in a healing way is much more difficult without the support of a counsellor.

During my counselling relationship with June, I almost exclusively concentrated on 'following' June empathically. Although this partly reflects my personal counselling style, I know that with other clients I do work differently and there will be much more of a focus upon a dynamic interaction between us. June did not need, at that time, to 'analyse' herself, to engage deeply with the dynamics between us or even to 'go to the real depths' of all her feelings. She was, at the time, struggling not to be consumed by her feelings and to develop a more secure sense of herself. She benefited greatly from a relationship where she could, increasingly, be herself without fear of judgement and where she knew she would be met with acceptance and understanding. She also benefited from the consistency and stability offered over time within that relationship. June had awareness of her feelings, was able and willing to share them and already had some inner capacity for personal reflection (there are many clients for whom none of those statements are true), but she could not do this work alone.

We should be careful not to overestimate the value of counselling but we should not underestimate it either. There can be no doubt that the love June has received from her husband, children, other family and friends has been far more important in her life than counselling ever could or should be. But at the same time, without receiving counselling at crucial times in her life, June might have been unable to receive or respond to that love. She might have been overcome by her devastating distress and rage, which so desperately needed to be heard. Looking back, June said to me that she is amazed she survived the ordeal of that particularly painful time when she came to see me. The pain was, she says, too much for her to have contained on her own—it was too overwhelming for her to cope with, she was simply 'in' it and in danger of being consumed by the distress and rage of it all. June says the sessions saved her from committing suicide and she may well be right. It is often my experience that when people are in acute distress the experience of being deeply heard and accepted provides a slender thread of hope which enables them to carry on during their most despairing moments. I remember a homeless young man who was only able to attend one and a half sessions, with a further, suicidal, session on the phone. I questioned the value of my limited work with him, and my own competence within it. Yet a whole year later, when he was once again in despair as a result of something very difficult that had happened he managed to find my number and call me again. He still wasn't ready to engage with an ongoing counselling relationship but our contact had clearly had an impact. When we are in deep despair the ability of another to acknowledge and receive our distress, to confirm and validate our being, is often sufficient to make the task of living once more seem worthwhile.

In my experience many people who have suffered greatly, when engaged with at depth, display considerable insight and awareness. June is one such person. I could speculate about how June gained this awareness. Perhaps it was from the previous counselling she had had some time before with a nun. Perhaps it was a natural, inborn capacity. Or perhaps it arose from a life in which suffering had forced her to look deeply

51

into herself—in some way a consequence of her trauma. This is an intriguing, if painful, possibility. Might suffering help us, sometimes, to be aware of the deeper levels of our experiencing and to consider our lives and how we live them more carefully?

We are all indelibly marked and changed by the tragedy that touches our lives. As June makes clear, the things that happened to her and the feelings they evoked will never leave her—they reach into the depths of her being and they are an important part of who she is and who she is becoming. We cannot erase these parts of her experience, though we might wish that they could have been prevented. We cannot take away her pain, though we can ensure that she does not have to bear it alone. We cannot remove her wounds but we can offer the time, understanding and tenderness that may enable these experiences to become less painful, less destructive and more integrated within her. So, now, June can say that she doesn't want the feelings to go away, because they are an important part of who she is and who she is becoming.

June's journey is ongoing and unfinished. Counselling is only a small part of that journey. Nevertheless it has helped June to be more able to live the life she chooses to live and be the person she wishes to be. She has become more sensitive to her own suffering and to the suffering of others; she has become more able to understand herself and to give and receive love; she is learning to accept all of herself and, in so doing, is becoming more able to accept others. Maybe the gift that suffering offers us is the opportunity to live more tenderly in the world.

REFERENCES

Larner, G (1999) Derrida and the deconstruction of power as context and topic in therapy. In I Parker (ed) *Deconstructing Psychotherapy* (pp. 39–53). London: Sage.

Rogers, CR (1959) A theory of therapy, personality, and interpersonal relationships, as developed in the client-centred framework. In S Koch (ed) *Psychology: A Study of Science, Vol. 3. Foundations of the person and the social context.* New York: McGraw-Hill.

Welwood, J (2000) *Toward a Psychology of Awakening: Buddhism, psychotherapy and the path of personal and spiritual transformation.* Boston: Shambhala.

CHAPTER 6

LOSS, LOVE AND MATERNAL DISTRESS

ELAINE CATTERALL

In the following case study I hope to demonstrate the place for positive growth in therapy, where 'cure' may not be possible in the context of the person's living circumstances. This was a very moving piece of work for me (and the client I believe), and validates for me, once again, the primacy of human relationships to our mental health and well-being. Elsewhere (Catterall, 2005), I have described in detail the theoretical aspects of counselling women experiencing maternal distress from a person-centred perspective, and therefore I encourage you to refer to this previous chapter for a more detailed discussion of maternal mental health and postnatal depression.

THE COUNSELLING SERVICE

One of my counselling contracts, with a local Sure Start project,[1] requires me to provide short-term individual counselling to parents who are registered with the project. The service is available to all parents, however only women have been referred for counselling so far. Most referrals come via Health Visitors and Sure Start workers who feel that individual counselling sessions will complement and add to the support services that are already being offered to the client. Because the counselling is a very limited service, it was agreed at the outset of my contract that an initial assessment meeting plus ten sessions would be the preferred service option.

This felt very uncomfortable at first as I had always been in the privileged position of offering open-ended counselling contracts to clients and this 'one size fits all' approach did not match my view of the idiosyncratic nature of the therapeutic process. However, working for such a worthwhile project, whose ideals for supporting women and their families resonate with mine, felt right and I realised that somehow I would have to become creative in my thinking and approach to the work. Indeed, I was soon to discover that ten sessions would simply not always be workable and on occasion I have been able to give an acceptable justification to the Sure Start team to extend the sessions. The client I have chosen represents such a case. (Whilst there are several women I could have

---

1. Sure Start is officially recognised as: 'the government programme set up to deliver the best start in life for every child, bringing together early education, childcare, health and family support'.

presented who experienced positive growth within the ten-session contract, the client I have chosen I met with for thirty-three sessions. The rationale for this extended contract will be explained below.)

MEETING JOSIE, AND THE COUNSELLING CONTRACT

A 27-year-old woman, whom I shall refer to as 'Josie' was seven months pregnant with her third child when she was referred for counselling by her health visitor. Josie was referred because of her very depressed and anxious state and the health visitor's concern about Josie's ability to cope with her other two pre-school children. Having left her children in the free crèche (situated opposite the counselling room), Josie came into the room and smiled at me fleetingly but became tearful almost as soon as she sat down.

Josie was overwhelmed by distress and sobbed all the while that she talked, putting me in mind of a young child who simply cannot contain their emotions. Any 'plan' I may have held before Josie's arrival about this being an assessment session and working through my brief assessment sheet in any kind of order, immediately went out of the window. This desperate young woman had me on the edge of my seat, engaged from the first moment and thrown right into her story, needing my absolute and full attention. I felt compassion and warmth for Josie and it seemed that we had embarked on an intense journey together without hesitation, before I had any time to reflect on the appropriateness of counselling for her.

In our first meeting I did, however, learn that she had moved back to the area to be near family and friends after separating (for the third time) from her abusive, alcoholic husband (whom I shall refer to as 'H'). Despite the practical support she was receiving from family and from Sure Start she felt isolated and lonely, and tensions were building with her parents because of what she perceived to be their interference in what 'help' she needed, particularly relating to how the children should be parented. She could not see how she would cope as a single mother, especially with another baby and the very real worry of being in huge financial debt. She felt powerless, with no sense of 'who I am anymore'. Importantly, she recognised her need to have time out from the children in order to be able to cope and that she wanted to use the counselling to 'talk about past experiences'.

Based on these aspects of Josie's story and her ability to engage with me I felt sure that the counselling could be useful to her but I also felt that ten sessions would not be enough, especially as the baby was due during this time, (and also knowing that the postnatal time for any woman can be a vulnerable time). I therefore took the decision to offer Josie an open-ended contract and explained my reasoning for this. Bearing in mind Josie's distressed state and sense of powerlessness, I think she would have agreed to anything in that moment so it felt important to explain my decision. The management at Sure Start were supportive of my judgement and we began working together immediately, keeping to a weekly meeting where possible.

FIVE SESSIONS BEFORE THE BABY ARRIVES

Working with any woman during the late stages of pregnancy is always a time of uncertainty from my perspective as the counsellor, because each session may be our last before the baby arrives. In some respects this parallels the woman's position as she grapples with the conflict of getting things prepared and ready, whilst thinking about the future and life with a new baby. With Josie, the time we had together before the birth felt like a rare opportunity to allow some time just to be with and experience the pregnancy. It transpired that this was something she had not done with this baby, and in fact described herself as 'being in denial' because this pregnancy was a reminder to her of the failings of her marriage. This baby was conceived shortly after Josie and H had reunited following an earlier separation. H's reaction to this pregnancy was the final insult to Josie when he accused her of having an affair and denounced the baby as 'not his'. To her, this somehow felt like a final act of betrayal—and unforgivable. Josie moved back to her home town almost immediately and started divorce proceedings, something she had never done before. Being able to confide her disconnection from and negativity about this third child without being judged brought some relief to Josie and, paradoxically, by bringing the baby 'into mind', connected her to the baby before the birth.

I am aware that I was working with an agenda during these sessions as I tend to do with all pregnant women, holding the possibility that an exploration of the woman's relationship with her unborn child (positive and negative) may help to clarify expectations about what the birth of this child may represent to the woman at this point in her life. I believe that the birth of each child will bring different hopes, fears and expectations reflecting where she is in her self-concept as a woman and as a mother.

The pregnancy was not the only focus for Josie during these sessions, however. Josie also started talking about the impact of the abusive relationship with H on her self-worth, as well as her fears for the effect it may have had on the children, particularly her son. This was very distressing for her to talk about and carried with it a deep sense of shame and guilt, feelings which made it even more difficult for her to cope with her son when he was 'being naughty'. Even during these early sessions Josie did demonstrate an ability to regain some power in her situation by deciding to involve a solicitor in relation to H requesting contact with the children. It was vital that I stayed very close to her story, listening and reflecting without passing judgement and, most importantly at this early stage in out relationship, keeping a sense of containment and safety. Whilst the person-centred practitioner may take this aspect of relating as fundamental to the therapeutic process, I point this out because I know that my personal style can be to move too quickly to focused exploration, which may have been too intense for Josie, especially so close to the birth. I also raise the (important) issue of safety and containment in relation to domestic abuse, as a sense of safety will have been absent from the marital relationship (Herman, 1992; Radford and Hester, 2006).

In these early sessions, a trusting relationship was established that enabled us to reconnect after a four-week break following the birth of the baby.

SESSION 6: THE SESSION FOLLOWING THE BIRTH

I am always preoccupied by a client's approaching birth when we are out of contact, waiting to hear, wondering how it will be for them. The Sure Start team informed me when Josie's baby was born and a week later updated me that the baby was ill and in hospital. Having to wait for Josie to contact me was difficult because of the background information I had been given. However, that had been our agreement so I waited for her call. She asked to see me via her outreach worker and we met a month after the birth of the baby.

Josie arrived with her month-old son, both looking surprisingly well. I commented on this. I think my expression of surprise revealed my own expectations that she would be looking 'worn out'—saying more about how I imagine I would have seemed following a new baby being ill. Josie felt relieved not to be pregnant any more as she had felt so physically restricted towards the end and so now felt better able to cope practically with the demands of three small children. Meeting her for the first time as a non-pregnant woman was also striking in that she sounded and seemed more able and in control. She had a different energy and a feisty determination about her, and also a smile; different from the sad and distressed young woman I had met two months earlier. (I was soon to discover however, that her smile was a deceptive mask at times.)

Whilst talking about the birth though, Josie became tearful when thinking about the baby being ill and being rushed to hospital, and this then triggered feelings of guilt and anxiety that her negativity and resentment towards the baby during the pregnancy had somehow caused the baby's illness. Allowing Josie the space to bring these fears into the open without 'rescuing' her from her guilt helped her to get in touch with a deeper, spiritual feeling quite new to Josie. For her, this experience was very uncomfortable as she faced the negative feelings that had surrounded the conception and arrival of her third child while at the same time experiencing her strong attachment and love for this child whom she thought might die. Josie had not followed any religion in a formal sense before, but had been moved spiritually by the experience, describing it as 'something bigger' than her, that had for the first time given her the opportunity to appreciate the preciousness of life, and to be thankful that she did in fact have her three children. This felt a very special moment that Josie shared, and which stood out from her past trauma and difficulties as a beacon of hope for the possibility of something different. There was no way of knowing whether this would be a fleeting experience for her, but I held onto the importance, within me, that this glimpse of 'something other' may bring with it the possibility of a different future for Josie, particularly as a mother but also as a young woman. This was an emotional session for Josie, which I also felt moved by. It left me feeling positive about her, and for her.

SESSIONS 7–23: COPING WITH THE PRESENT WHILST EXPLORING THE PAST

This phase of the therapy was very much about the current difficulties that Josie faced adjusting to life as a single parent and also the challenges that this presented in terms of her attitudinal beliefs about herself and others. This meant that during the sessions there was a constant weaving together of present and past experiences.

I will now briefly outline the issues that were explored in these sessions and then I shall consider the main themes that emerged.

Feelings of depression and anxiety surfaced again, as though the early postnatal bubble of energy and hope had dissipated. Josie did not want to admit these feelings to anyone for fear of being judged as not coping as a mother; however, she said it was a relief to share them with me. These feelings also reminded her of her experience of postnatal depression following the birth of her first child and this brought back painful memories of that time in her life when she was lonely, living away from her home town and beginning to realise that her marriage was not good. The thought of sinking into postnatal depression again really frightened her as it felt different somehow to depression she had felt at other times (an observation made by many women experiencing postnatal depression).[2] In session eight she described feeling 'sucked dry' by everyone and that if she didn't get any space she'd 'self-destruct'. The enormity of her situation was overwhelming her and by the end of this session I too felt swamped and hopeless that Josie's life could ever improve.

Over the coming weeks, the stress of her living conditions (a cramped, damp, two-bedroomed council flat), increasing tensions with her parents trying to 'take over' her life, and ongoing anxieties and uncertainties about the baby's health made it almost impossible for Josie to focus on anything positive.

The only thing that she could look forward to, it seemed, was the possibility of an improvement in the quality of her daily living when rehoused. (A letter from me to the housing office in support of Josie's need for rehousing on mental health grounds was responded to promptly and did appear to accelerate the process.) Although the house move was wanted, it added greatly to the tensions and stress running between Josie and her parents, and by session sixteen she was overwhelmed and worn out by it all.

Alongside the daily stresses and current difficulties she was experiencing, Josie was also exploring the relationship with her ex-husband, who had moved back to the local area. The occasional glimpse of him or a member of his family would trigger the rage and hurt she felt about how he had treated her in the past and about his present apparent lack of interest and concern for the children, particularly the baby's health. The thought that she and the children did not matter to him or his family was unbearable, leaving her feeling unloved and unlovable.

Interestingly, as much as Josie tried to push him from her mind, those around her always seemed to want to tell her what he had been up to, perpetuating his presence in her life. Therefore, some of the work in therapy looked at varying ways that Josie could

2. For further consideration of maternal depression see Catterall (2005).

cope with these unwanted and unhelpful intrusions and explored her style of communication to see what impact this may be having on such conversations. This was directive, and a diversion away from staying with her experiencing into teaching communication and assertiveness skills. Yet it was helpful to her and, whilst she did not want to hear about him, it did reveal that she still felt attached to H and was still living in hope of him changing and of things working out between them.

In session seventeen, Josie was tearful and described feeling depressed, yet for the first time she had done something quite different with these difficult feelings outside of the therapy: she had confided her true feelings about 'everything' to an old friend and, to her surprise and relief, this friend had been very accepting. This reconnected Josie to several relationships that had, in fact, been important to her since childhood and signalled the start of her seeking support from people outside of her immediate family.

SHAME AND GRIEF

The two major feeling states that weaved through Josie's story are shame and grief. These both appeared repeatedly, sometimes separate, sometimes intertwined, and were expressed both within the content of the narrative and directly by her feelings and behaviour. By staying with, and accepting, these parts of Josie I attempted to provide her with a safe, non-judgemental space in which to approach distressing feelings and memories. With respect to shameful experiences and feelings, Josie started to shift from a place of relational isolation associated with the shame process to a place of relational support; firstly with me and, increasingly, with friends as the therapy progressed.

Josie suffered many losses associated with her marriage and with motherhood and gradually she was able to really bring her anger and sadness about these into the room, feelings she had previously tried to avoid, either by believing she should just 'get on with it', or by misdirecting them towards the children.

The impact of shame and loss on Josie's sense of self will become evident within the themes that follow.

CONDITIONS OF WORTH, THE MYTH OF THE FAIRY-TALE MARRIAGE, AND BEING A SINGLE PARENT

A key theme that emerged in metaphor in the first session and weaved its way throughout out time together was that of the 'fairy-tale romance', as she described it, where she had married her 'Prince' and assumed they would live 'happily ever after'. When she filed for divorce this fairy tale started to fall apart and the thought of being a single mother was unbearable and shameful to Josie.

Josie's feelings and beliefs about marriage become more meaningful when they are considered within the context of the family discourse that she grew up with. The fairy tale of 'living happily ever after' in marriage seems to be the narrative held by her parents whom she perceived as being ashamed of their daughter for not staying in the marriage for 'the sake of the children'. Josie described how they consider the traditional family set-up to be the only socially accepted (respectable) tradition in which to bring up children. Therefore, to the outside world they must be seen to be a 'happy family' and any discord within the family must stay within the family so as not to bring judgement or shame from outside. Trying to live within this narrative only served to isolate Josie in her experience, preventing her from sharing her emotional difficulties and vulnerabilities which she felt would not be accepted because 'Josie had made her bed and she should lie in it'. Reflecting on this theme in supervision gave me some insight into Josie's fierce determination 'to cope alone' in order to feel in control of her life but also highlighted an association for her that support (from her parents) meant not coping (i.e. failing).

In the first session Josie showed her distress about this fairy-tale ending and her sense of shame and failure, but as the sessions progressed and she started to regain control over her life. She was able to reflect more realistically on the abusive aspects of the marital relationship, start to deconstruct the myth of the fairy-tale marriage and to acknowledge that it was not all about her 'being a failure'. With this came a growing (but fragile) sense of self-worth which was reflected in Josie starting to value her own needs; for example, starting to accept social invitations from friends, organise babysitters and take more care and interest in her appearance.

However, her changing self-concept, combined with a growing internal locus of evaluation, began to conflict with, and diverge from, the views of her parents. This triggered ambivalent feelings of frustration and anger relating to her need for autonomy and acceptance whilst at the same time she experienced feelings of anxiety about her need to be approved of as a 'good daughter' and 'mother' by her parents. Using the space in therapy to explore the increasing external pressure and criticism she faced from her parents, particularly from her mother, whilst holding on to and validating her own experiencing, enabled Josie to gain some insight into those 'family values' that had formed a part of her conditions of worth and had served to perpetuate the shame she felt about 'failing' in her marriage, 'failing' as a mother to protect the children from their abusive father, and even 'failing' to provide her children with a good enough father in the first place. As long as Josie felt a sense of powerlessness in her relationships such feelings would be triggered by perceived disapproval and would come up again in the therapy.

THE IMPACT OF DOMESTIC VIOLENCE

There is plenty of documented evidence (e.g. Herman, 1992; Radford and Hester, 2006) that domestic violence and abuse entraps women in relationships where personal power and autonomy, as well as self-worth, are eroded. Leaving an abusive partner is a complex decision and often puts the woman at risk of further assault following separation. Additionally, taking children away from their father makes the decision to leave even harder.

Josie talked about her relationship with H frequently, describing distressing incidents in detail, sometimes becoming upset and tearful, but mostly becoming angry. However, it seemed that expressing anger was only part of the therapeutic process for Josie as it often felt as if we were circling the same known terrain, with Josie talking about her need to 'move on and forget him. Why should I be the one who is upset and suffering?' and yet ... what else was she experiencing? In writing such a statement, I feel I am in danger of trivialising what is a traumatic story; however, what I want to convey is my sense of something 'other' (something at the edge of my awareness) as I stayed with her, circling around in the anger that was certainly very real and present. In session fifteen, Josie shared her fury and hurt at discovering H was expecting another child with his new girlfriend. Her pity for this other woman and her anger at his lack of responsibility seemed to be part of her self-protective process to avoid her own painful feelings. In the next few sessions this latest blow left her too tired and broken to see any way forward so in session eighteen I suggested using a sheet of paper to express all her feelings about H. (I never have an agenda for directive interventions of this type but sometimes it feels OK to offer an alternative way to explore something.)

Josie was up for this and set about producing a spider diagram (a positive spin-off of this exercise was how it reminded her of the skills she had gained during her working career) which clearly articulated the full impact of H's abusive behaviour on her own self-confidence but also highlighted to her what an abusive father he had been, particularly to their young son. Josie's complete incomprehension and anger at his behaviour emerged as she talked through this diagram; also her deep shame about being with a 'man like that' and guilt at not having left him sooner because of the way he treated their son. Although it was a distressing exercise, because it showed Josie much of what she had lost in her life and within herself, it did help to validate for her why she was 'right' to have finally left. She lost her career and financial security when she married and was left with many of H's heavy debts (all in her name). Facing the shame and anger she felt about this moved her to take the decision to declare herself bankrupt: an uncomfortable decision but a solution all the same.

Apart from the children (who, for Josie, were the one mixed blessing amongst all that had gone wrong), she really felt as though she was starting her life 'all over again'.

SPIRITUALITY:
THE PRESENCE OF SOMETHING 'BIGGER THAN US'

I described how, in session six, Josie's anxiety about the baby's health following the birth had moved her to a level of spiritual reflection completely new to her. This experience proved not to be fleeting, as Josie chose to act on this by having all three children christened. This symbolised Josie's appreciation of the preciousness of life and represented a way to offer something new and 'good' to her children as well as bringing herself and her children into the wider community of the church. Just as significantly I think, it provided Josie with a formal way to include a wider circle of adults into her children's lives by way of godparents.

SESSIONS 24–30: GRIEVING, LETTING GO, AND ENDINGS

In session twenty-four Josie cried, for the first time, for the good things she missed about H. She admitted that she had been too scared up to this point to acknowledge any good aspects of their relationship for fear that any positive memories would suggest enough reason to go back to him. I was also left wondering whether it was only now in our relationship that she felt safe enough to explore this more hidden aspect of self, trusting that I would be able to accept that part of her that wanted to return to an abusive relationship, the part of her that others just couldn't understand and judged harshly. Whatever the reason, this session proved to be very significant in terms of Josie's exploration of her previous relationships with men and her attitude to sex and intimacy. She spoke for the first time (to anyone) about how she had been sexually assaulted at fourteen by a boy who then spread rumours at school, resulting in Josie being bullied for being a 'slag'. This was deeply distressing for Josie to share. During these moments in therapy I am aware how quietly attentive I become, in my body and my communications, as if too much of my presence at such moments would trample on or distract a client from their fragile processing, yet all the while feeling as if this is the most important thing I must listen and bear witness to in order to catch every word and meaning.

Following this disclosure, Josie started to reflect on how this first traumatic, sexual experience and the subsequent name calling, had coloured her view of herself as being a sexual object to men and how she then started to live by her 'reputation'; becoming sexually promiscuous and reckless, preferring one-night (drunken) stands to long-term relationships, as she thought this was what men wanted. She also realised that becoming pregnant early on in her relationship with H removed her need to make a choice about committing to marriage—the pregnancy decided that for her. Reflecting on her previous sexual relationships highlighted to Josie that, whilst this behaviour had given her a sense of control in relationships, she had been refusing to care for herself or take responsibility for her actions. Recently, however, she had acted differently when out with friends. She had drunk too much and was heading home with some guy but said 'goodnight' at the door rather than letting him stay the night. Josie described this as being 'completely out of character' but, in the light of our exploration, it signalled how she wanted relationships with men to be different now.

Following this, and the next four sessions, Josie reflected on and cried a lot about her relationship with H. Much of this grief process was occurring between sessions and what it highlighted to Josie was that, although she wanted to move on and focus on the future, she couldn't until she felt the relationship had really ended. She wasn't sure what this actually meant to her though.

During this time, the mother of a close friend died suddenly: a woman that Josie described as a 'second Mum', someone she had been close to since childhood and whom she felt was more understanding than her own mother. I was concerned for Josie that this bereavement could be a major setback to her, yet the effect it seemed to have was a positive one in that it showed her that she was in fact emotionally strong enough to support her bereaved friend, and it brought a level of intimacy back to their relationship which had faded when Josie had married and moved away.

The theme of endings seemed ever present for Josie during these sessions and was starting to create anxiety for me about Josie's dependency on the counselling. Although our contract was open-ended I was also aware of my growing waiting list and the conflict I had of trying to remain with Josie's experiencing whilst being aware of an increasing urgency to direct our work towards an ending. I had in fact introduced the idea of endings as early as session fifteen—a possibility which, as she showed by her anxious, agitated and negative response, was unbearable to Josie at the time. As the sessions progressed though, it was an issue that was increasingly present within the therapy room; in terms of her process of mourning what was lost, and in terms of the therapeutic relationship being finite.

SESSIONS 29 AND 30: THE SPELL IS BROKEN

During the week Josie saw H sitting outside a local pub with a pint of beer at 11a.m. She described this chance sighting as the moment that 'broke the spell' for her of him ever changing: when she realised that his love for alcohol was greater than his love for her and the children. The fairy-tale romance was finally over. She realised that this was what she had been waiting for; somehow seeing the reality of his life clearly, without the distorting lens of false hope she had been clinging to (that he cared enough about her to change). She did not become distressed as she described this event. There was an air of anger as she recounted this story but Josie was being much more self-reflective in this session, thinking about the future and what she wanted for herself. In contrast to earlier sessions she was starting to think about the future in terms of herself as a single person, rather than in terms of herself needing to have a partner and this was a significant turning point for Josie in her self-valuing process.

In the following session, Josie described feeling anxious and panicky. She had bumped into H, almost literally, whilst shopping, only this time she felt unprepared and unsafe in his presence. No words were exchanged, only glances. We used this session to focus on how she might handle similar situations in the future so that she felt more 'prepared' and this helped Josie contain her anxiety about facing him when alone, especially with the children. Despite this 'setback', Josie for the first time suggested an ending date for the counselling. My feeling inside was one of elation and validation that, yet again, by trusting the client's process the move from dependency to autonomy within the therapeutic relationship will happen. (I was also relieved that I did not have to impose an ending!)

SESSIONS 31–33: RECONNECTING WITH OLD FRIENDS AS A BRIDGE TO THE FUTURE

In session thirty-one Josie arrived buzzing with excitement because an old friend was visiting from abroad and the experience of reconnecting with her past, single life helped her to see how far she had come and how well she was coping now. She realised that for the first time in several years she was able to laugh and share in the joking banter, and she was enjoying rediscovering her humorous side. She felt able to tell this friend 'everything' about the domestic violence and the reality of her life when she was married. This was an important step for Josie because she was starting to begin the task of breaking the silence about the domestic abuse, something that she had been too ashamed to do previously. The friend's visit provided Josie with a link back to a time when she had been happier and more self-confident and this, interestingly, became a bridge to her future as they met up with old friends and work colleagues. Josie had not realised how well-liked and respected she was by them and, although it was uncomfortable disclosing some of her experiences to this wider circle, she could now understand why people needed to know something of her past to be able to fill in the 'gaps' and make sense of where she was now.

Josie said she felt this was the first time in counselling that she had nothing she needed to talk about! I could only respond to such a statement with an observation that it seemed then, that only the negative, rather than positive aspects of our lives need to be 'talked about' in counselling, yet the positive aspects explored in this session seemed just as important because they clearly showed how much she was changing and developing in terms of her self-awareness and increasing ability to take responsibility for her life! I find it so fascinating that the positive aspects of change can be so easily incorporated into a client's life without then stopping to notice; aspects that are so significant, yet almost missed or taken for granted.

A final task that Josie undertook in terms of separating further from H was to write a letter to him (something she had mentioned several times previously). This was something she now felt able to do and brought it to the session. She did not want to read it to me as she felt it had been enough to write it. She felt angry as she wrote it but not so upset that she needed to cry—and that felt good. She tore it up in front of me (without it being read) and for her this symbolic action felt enough.

AGREEING TO END, AND REVIEWING THE COUNSELLING PROCESS

Due to the approaching summer holidays we suddenly found ourselves with only two more sessions together. (Josie suddenly decided she did not want to come back after a long summer break.) We reviewed Josie's process through therapy, although we had already started a spontaneous review in recent sessions.

Josie's review of the counselling process was that she now felt more self-confident and relaxed. She felt she knew herself better and had regained her sense of humour. She felt more able to take on adult responsibilities, which she summed up with the comment 'I've grown up'—and my thought in response to this was that yes, indeed, you are no longer 'a reckless teenager'.

REFLECTING ON MOTHERHOOD

As part of our final review I encouraged Josie to think about her role as a mother and how she now viewed herself in this role. When I first met Josie she felt overwhelmed and distressed about coping with her children, so how did she feel now? As I described earlier, the shock of the new baby's ill health had a huge impact on Josie and her view of the preciousness of life. However, as we looked back together over the first seven month's of the baby's life, Josie was able to acknowledge how the frequent readmissions to hospital had heightened her fear of not knowing what was really going on and not trusting that the baby would be OK. This fear had been reflected in earlier sessions in terms of her anxiety about being able to cope when the baby was ill, as well as in her sense of powerlessness and frustration with the doctors for not being able to give her a definitive diagnosis. As she reflected on this experience, she described how she had started to see the baby as separated into 'the baby' and 'the illness', whereas now she was starting to enjoy the baby more and view the illness as a part of his whole person. Josie had found it difficult to admit to this detachment a few months earlier because of the guilt she was experiencing. From a theoretical perspective I was hearing how the attachment relationship between Josie and the baby was disrupted and threatened by the baby's illness and how important it was, therefore, for Josie to be able to explore the impact of the baby's illness on their relationship without fear of judgement.

With respect to her other two children, much of the early focus had been around her fears about the effects of the marital relationship on her eldest son and her own subsequent difficulties in coping with his 'naughty' behaviour. Now, however, she felt better able to cope alone and in fact felt very strongly that she did not want this stability disrupted by their father. When we explored this further she felt that all the while H's behaviour stayed the same, he was not fit as a father and she would not let him see the children. When I asked her whether she thought living with domestic violence had affected her abilities as a mother, she said that she felt she actually had more time for the children now as a single parent because she was less preoccupied and anxious about 'what H would do next'. She enjoys them now in a way she never could before. This aspect of Josie's lived experience really challenged my attitudes and beliefs about children always benefiting from continued access to both parents following separation. With further reading (e.g. Radford and Hester, 2006; Golombeck, 2000) I realised that Josie was right to trust her internal valuing process on this issue and felt humbled by her courage to fight for what she felt was best for her children, even though denying H access to the children goes against the current philosophy of the family legal system.

CONDITIONAL ACCEPTANCE AND BLOCKS TO EMPATHY

The greatest challenge for me when I explore the theme of parenting with clients is when their parenting styles and beliefs differ greatly from mine. At times Josie would talk very harshly and negatively about her children's behaviour and describe responses that showed little empathy for them. At such times I know I found it difficult to experience her unconditionally, withdrawing from her frame of reference into imagining what that experience might be like for her children. When I retreated like this, back into my own frame (and my empathy and acceptance for her were lost), I was aware of wanting to become directive by trying to get Josie to imagine the experience from the children's point of view. Whilst this may have been helpful at times, it might also have been unhelpful and counter-therapeutic if I had taken it to another level where an exploratory challenge becomes authoritative advice-giving and where a perceived loss of empathy from me could have left Josie feeling negatively judged as a mother. The fact that this work is set within a multidisciplinary setting is enormously helpful in dealing with such conflicting issues because I knew that Josie had requested, and was receiving, help with her skills in managing the children's challenging behaviour so I did not need to dwell on this important, but separate, issue of parenting skills. Whilst Josie had a somewhat harsh, no-nonsense attitude towards managing the children, she also had a wonderfully soft and imaginatively playful side which the children also benefited from, so if our work together had got bogged down in how she could 'improve' her parenting skills, it may have overshadowed a celebration of what she was doing so well already.

SAYING GOODBYE

Our last session felt like a 'good' ending for both of us and that the 'work' she had set out to do was finished. The session was kept light-hearted, littered with laughter and smiles rather than tears. Josie said she felt OK about ending and wanted to keep looking forward now. She had ideas of going to night-school to learn something new and eventually head back to work. We talked about the option of a follow-up session, which Josie thought would be good 'but not too soon—give me at least nine months!' That time is nearly upon us and I wonder with curiosity how she will respond to such an invitation.

PERSON-CENTRED THERAPY: A SUCCESSFUL MODEL FOR FACILITATING CONSTRUCTIVE PSYCHOLOGICAL GROWTH

I have no doubt about the successful outcome of this piece of therapeutic work. Josie clearly demonstrated positive psychological growth through the process of therapy, becoming more open to, and less afraid of, her authentic subjective experiencing, which in turn resulted in a growing sense of self-regard and acceptance, and a greater emotional stability. Constructive psychological change was also evident in her rediscovery of positive qualities and talents (e.g. sense of humour, playfulness, organisational skills). As the therapeutic relationship strengthened, Josie engaged in the process with a courage and determination that empowered her to recognise the importance of her own agency and the need to start taking personal responsibility for life decisions.

The person-centred theory of constructive personality change in psychotherapy (Rogers, 1959) is founded on the assumption that human beings have an inherent tendency towards growth, development and optimal functioning. However, as Rogers stated, to actualise this inherent potential a person needs to experience the right social environment, and in terms of the therapeutic relationship providing such an environment, Rogers described *six necessary and sufficient conditions* of the therapy relationship to promote therapeutic personality change (Rogers, 1957). Against this theoretical background, and from personal experience, I do believe that it is the relational nature of our experiences that promotes or hinders our inherent capacity for psychological growth, love and to live more meaningful and satisfying lives. And crucially, such experiences are not static, as our social (relational) environment is subject to change and new possibilities. Therefore, just as destructive relational experiences can harm our self-concept, well-being and psychological growth, constructive relationships can provide the opportunity for healing and growth.

From the outset Josie was ready to engage with me psychologically and for my part I was able to bring myself authentically into the relationship with the *necessary* attitudinal qualities to facilitate psychological exploration, insight and growth in Josie.

To witness the actualising tendency at work within Josie in terms of her increasingly pro-social behaviour and psychological growth (see Rogers, 1961 or Merry, 2004 for an overview), as well as to hear her 'living in the moment' as she started to recount experiences of being spontaneously playful in relationships, was truly inspiring and moving for me and I felt privileged to be a part of a relationship that had a significant part to play in one woman's process of growing self-awareness and healing.

COMPARING THE MEDICAL MODEL CONCEPT OF 'CURE' WITH THE POSITIVE PSYCHOLOGY MODEL OF PROMOTING 'THE GOOD LIFE'

If I evaluated this work against the medical model for mental illness I would have to think in terms of diagnosis, treatment and cure. Had the 'talking cure' worked as a form of treatment? Symptoms associated with Josie's feelings of depression and anxiety had lessened by the end of the therapy and she was no longer overwhelmed by her distress. She was happier. I do not believe, however, that Josie would never feel anxious or depressed again when:

• she continues to live with the uncertainty and anxiety about the children's well-being and the baby's health in particular;
• she is learning to live with the financial stresses associated with being a single parent supported by state benefit payments;

- she continues to cope with three small children without the emotional support of a loving, caring partner.

For me, the concept of 'cure' for psychological distress is unhelpful and meaningless when a person's lived experience continues to be informed by such challenging social constraints. What seems more pertinent in relation to reducing psychological distress is that, despite the limitations of her social life space (Mearns and Thorne, 2000), Josie has found (through the therapeutic relationship) more meaningful and personally fulfilling ways to live. Can we ask for more than that?

REFERENCES

Catterall, E (2005) Working with maternal depression: Person-centred therapy as part of a multidisciplinary approach. In S Joseph and R Worsley (eds) *Person-Centred Psychopathology. A positive psychology of mental health* (pp. 202–25). Ross-on-Wye: PCCS Books.

Golombeck, S (2000) *Parenting: What really counts.* London: Routledge.

Herman, JI (1992) *Trauma and Recovery: From domestic abuse to political violence.* London: Pandora.

Mearns, D and Thorne, B (2000) *Person-Centred Therapy Today: New frontiers in theory and practice.* London: Sage.

Merry, T (2004) Classical client-centred therapy. In P Sanders (ed) *The Tribes of the Person-Centred Nation* (pp. 2–44). Ross-on-Wye: PCCS Books.

Radford, L and Hester, M (2006) *Mothering through Domestic Violence.* London: Jessica Kingsley.

Rogers, CR (1957) The necessary and sufficient conditions of therapeutic personality change. *Journal of Consulting Psychology, 2,* 95–103.

Rogers, CR (1959) A theory of therapy, personality, and interpersonal relationships, as developed in the client-centred framework. In S Koch (ed) *Psychology: A Study of a Science, Vol. 3. Formulations of the person and the social contract.* New York: McGraw-Hill.

CHAPTER 7

THE BARNEY BAG:
A TACIT VARIABLE IN THE
THERAPEUTIC RELATIONSHIP

JEROLD D. BOZARTH AND ANN GLAUSER

> I have been looking in my Barney Bag
> And I found a lot of things.
> Gizmos and gadgets and odds and ends,
> And even some old string.
> So let's ask ourselves the question
> What can we make today?
> With imagination and the Barney Bag
> We will see what we can make today.
>
> *The Barney Bag* (song from the 1994 video, *Barney Live*)

Most psychotherapists need a Barney Bag from time to time. In most psychotherapy the Barney Bag might represent systematic 'interventions' that are premised on the notion of the 'specificity myth' (Bozarth, 1998, 2002); namely, that there are viable specific treatments for specific dysfunction (e.g. psychoanalytic, behavioral). Other psychotherapies have in their bag systematic processes to help their clients to become more connected with inner processes (e.g. experiential, person-centered, focusing-oriented therapies).

Client-centered therapy (Rogers, 1959) offers the only model that creates psychological freedom for the client to find her direction and process in her own way. Even aspects of client-centered therapy might restrict the client's opportunities to go in her own direction, way and pace. For example, response repertoire, ('reflection', 'reflection of feeling', 'empathic understanding responses') as a systematic response system can also become part of the 'Barney Bag' phenomena. Systematic and unspecified activities and responses primarily provide the therapist with a sense of security and may not thwart the direction of the client if the therapist sincerely trusts the client.

In any case, it is the client/therapist relationship and not the theory of therapy that dictates the therapist's trust of the client (Rogers, 1957) and it is the relationship and client resources that account for most of the variance for therapeutic success (Lambert, 1992). In short, it is the therapist's attitude, and particularly the trust in the client's capacities, rather than a particular system of therapy that determines the extent of trust in the client. The fundamental therapeutic assumptions of client-centered therapy are, in our assessment, more directly associated with this trust.

The rise of positive psychology compels us to embrace psychotherapy that leads individuals to experience a sense of well-being and meaningfulness while alleviating impediments to happiness. Our therapeutic bias is one that fits the paradigm of a positive psychology. It is from this stance that we decided to examine our interactions with two individuals. (The interactions with one individual are presented here.) Perhaps the most personal might prove to be the most universal. To us, a positive psychotherapy would:

• assist a person to hold fewer conditions of worth,
• find a high level of psychological adjustment, and
• enable a person to be increasingly aware of their values and feelings.

Accomplishing these goals increases the individual's capacity to resolve her problems and diminish dysfunction, and constructive personality change results in greater capacity to resolve problems and reduce dysfunction.

Our inquiry into a client's experience of her therapy involves a therapist (also referred to as counselor) who had the intent of creating freedom for the client to develop self-determination and discover self-resources. Her Barney Bag consists of a wide array of unsystematic and spontaneous reflections congruent with her unconditional reception of the client. The therapist's focus is on the client's world, with the assumption that such trust enables the client to become more self-determined and 'fully functioning'.

THE COUNSELING / SUPERVISION EXPERIENCE

The therapist (Ann) e-mailed two previous clients, last contacted over four months ago, about the possibility of meeting first with her and then with her supervisor. The purpose of meeting with the supervisor was to provide feedback on their experience with Ann. Both clients agreed. They were informed that the sessions would be audio-taped, but that the tape recorder could be turned off at any time during their feedback session with Jerry (Jerold). Neither client requested that the recorder be turned off at any time. Both signed an informed consent giving Ann and Jerry permission to tape. The university research protocol procedures were followed. Consistent with standard ethical practice, the tapes have been destroyed and portions of the transcriptions of the meetings have been deleted rendering them useless for recovery of identifiers provided by the clients. Rather large sections of the transcribed session with Ann were deleted due to identifying details (i.e. names, places of employment and schools attended) to preserve the anonymity of the clients. We believe that the abbreviated session reported with Ann that eliminates identifying details of the client's life is adequate because the intent of this chapter is to capture the clients' experiences with Ann.

Only the first client is presented in this chapter. The second client session and interview were examined in the same manner but not included in this chapter. Our general conclusions about the second client were consistent with the conclusions presented in this chapter. The interviewer had no prior knowledge about the clients.

GUIDING PRINCIPLES OF THE THERAPIST (ANN)

Clients are generally referred to me, or self-referred, for specific reasons. They often come to me with the expectation that I will help them to find practical solutions or obtain pragmatic suggestions to deal effectively with a specific concern related to academics (i.e. writing or test anxiety, motivation, procrastination, or selecting a major). However, I might do many things that emerge out of my relationship with the client. This might be part of the reason that I have, what I metaphorically call, a 'Barney Bag' that I reach for when individuals consistently ask for something. Although I don't believe I have ever found an opportunity to pull any 'string' from my 'bag', I have pulled some 'gizmos and gadgets and odds and ends' such as specific information, suggestions, songs, books, poems, other people, and my own experiences. These items that I reach for are spontaneous and not designed or predetermined prior to the session. The effectiveness of my therapy is based upon the relationship that forms between the client and me and is not so much related to what *I do* in the counseling session that provides for a positive experience for the client. How *I am* in the relationship is the essential element for me. Even though I may offer suggestions from my own experiences when I feel obligated or insecure, I have a profound trust in the client's self-directive variables and in their capacity to deal with their life context. I strive to follow the necessary and sufficient conditions of client-centered therapy in an effort to create a facilitative space for my client. Once this space is created I feel free to be with the client and begin by encouraging the client to be free with me, which includes rejecting any suggestions from my Barney bag.

GUIDING PRINCIPLES OF THE INTERVIEWER (JERRY)

As a therapist, my intention is to follow the instructions of client-centered therapy as depicted in Rogers' (1959: 213) chapter. Functionally, my focus is upon:
- maximizing my trust in the clients' inherent capacities to direct their own lives,
- directing my attention solely upon what the world is like for the particular person, and
- being aware of what I am experiencing during a session.

My Barney Bag refers to the things that I do during my interaction in the client's world. As an interviewer, my intention is similar to that of being in a therapeutic relationship. However, I am likely to have particular questions and to say or do some things that I would be unlikely to say or do in a therapy session.

EXAMINATION OF THE THERAPY SESSION AND INTERVIEW

A retrospect coding by the authors follows most of the responses of the therapist and the interviewer. This was a post-hoc decision after we decided that some of our responses might interrupt the client's direction. The notations are identified by the following code:

I = *Interruptive*. This indicates that the client, Berdie, responds in a way that the response redirected her thoughts.

NI = *Non-Interruptive*. This indicates that the client seemed to either ignore or to use the response to continue in her own direction. The therapist and interviewer present some of the thoughts and experiences that they remember at any given time.

THE SESSION (Reported by the therapist)

Berdie, the client, first met with me during her third semester of college. Her initial request was that I help her get back on track academically. She expressed concerns that she was disorganized (particularly with studying), and that she often found herself procrastinating. At the same time she lacked motivation to complete academic tasks due to medical conditions that exhausted her physically. We met six or seven times throughout the semester. At her request, I pulled from my Barney Bag practical advice for managing time and organizing learning materials.

Therapy session

(The therapist's thoughts are presented in this typeface)

Berdie: [Sneeze. Sneeze. Sneeze.] *I am always cold. I broke down and took some medication, but my body didn't handle it.* [Sneeze.] *I have so much stuff to do. It's stressful and then on top of that, I have been having blood sugar issues again. I do eat, but just not enough. I need to eat more because I am doing a lot more in the day, and it's just real frustrating.*

Ann: When did it change? NI

I am thinking that I need to check to determine if she has gone to a new doctor or nutritionist.

Berdie: My whole body aches. I can feel it.

Ann: So it's not only all the stuff on the outside that is coming at you, but in trying to get things done, it's also inside your body running rampant. NI

I feel this glop running quickly through her body that is stuffing her up, stagnating her. I visualize buzzing bees all around her, preventing her from moving forward.

Berdie: Yeah. I'm trying to take tests, trying to get things done. In class, the teacher is trying to put the organization on us ... organization is not my forte. She is disorganized and wants us to analyze, think on a higher order and a lower order. Normally teachers just give you all the information and you have to take it and turn it into something more substantial.

Ann: You have to search for the organization in her disorganization. NI

I visualize Berdie sitting in a large lecture class trying to focus, trying to sift through all the information presented. Again I see bees buzzing around her.

71

Berdie: She pretty much gives you the information, but sometimes ... for example, maybe once a week, she says, 'Here's an experiment. Tell me what they were trying to find'. We then have to pick apart the information by ourselves, which is very frustrating to me. But she is actually doing what teachers are suppose to be doing, but I am frustrated the way other students treat her, like talking during class. They can't handle her teaching style, her accent. They are rude to her. I am so ready to get out of undergraduate school, and I haven't even ... I am just starting my major. I want to do a double major and with one extra semester ... [The next three to four minutes of the tape produce garbled sounds. During this portion of the session, Berdie discussed her undergraduate and graduate plans as well as her desire to establish citizenship in another country. She mentions that she has talked with different people to find out what they have done and some of them have done things that are 'phenomenal'.] *I want to be feeling like I am doing something productive like earning money and working towards my overall cause. But all of it depends financially and stability-wise on how long I can handle being in school.*

Ann: You are ready to get on the path ... get going. NI

I think of the community-chest card in the game Monopoly that allows you to travel directly to Go and collect $200.

Berdie: I want to do some volunteer work experiences, but work towards being financially independent. I just get really overwhelmed because I am bad at breaking things down. I just want to do it all at once.

Ann: [The tape is pretty garbled. I ramble on for quite some time.] NI

What few words or phrases that can be picked up on the tape do not seem very insightful.

Berdie: On top of all this, at any given point, there are all these books around me. I start one, put it down, and start something else. I forget about it. Go to something different. It's not that I don't get anything from them. I just don't get that sense of completion.

Ann: So is that the story of your life? Involvement in so many things? I

Berdie: Yeah [halfheartedly] *... On the plus side, mother has been ridiculously busy so now we only talk about every three days.* [Berdie goes on to talk about disagreements her divorced parents have about financial matters concerning her.] *It is frustrating because of all the financial, medical complications.*

Ann: So you are looking for some relief. NI

I experience her wearing a backpack full of rocks while trying to walk up a hill.

Berdie: Well, my mother is. I put all the e-mails from my parents in a box to maybe read later. [She then goes on to talk more about her parent's conflicted relationship as well as her own with her father and the impending possibility of total estrangement with her father as a result of possible legal action. She also mentions that her wisdom teeth are coming in, but she has neither the time nor money to deal with them.]

Ann: There is a lot of stuff going on. Sometimes when you are talking about what this

person might do in reaction to this other person, it sounds like a weatherman forecasting a tornado that is coming. NI

I visualize a tornado coming towards her.

Berdie: I am late to everything. I am getting my schoolwork done, but last minute. Assignments are sneaking up on me. I have been putting off dealing with medical bills that Mom wants to send to her lawyer. I know it needs to be done.

Ann: It's frustrating knowing what your father's reaction will be. NI

I think of an explosion.

Berdie: It's more like pressing the red button.

Ann: It's going to be activated. NI

Berdie: It's not like me to put off a favor to mom. I am here; I am going through all of this shit, going through the motions at school, surrounded by a bunch of idiots. I am just trying to remind myself not to get disgruntled and keep working towards what I am working towards. It is disheartening to see what the bulk of middle-America is like. I can generally deal with drunken, stupid people, but lately I have seen so much of a consumer nation.

Ann: You are surrounded by all this crap ... NI

Berdie: And I am stepping forward. [She gives more examples of stupid people in class. She then talks about her speech on gypsies that she gave to the class.] *Gypsies observe a lot and only people within the group know them. Pretty much everywhere gypsies have gone they have been misunderstood, slandered, driven out of town.*

I visualize Berdie as a child, dressed as a gypsy. I feel like a grandmother.

Ann: You are like a gypsy sometimes. Watching, but not revealing or maybe that's just me. NI

Berdie: Yeah ...

Ann: I think of gypsies as being very astute in terms of watching and not revealing so much about themselves to people out there but within their group people probably know each other really well. NI

Berdie: Uh huh. [Silence] *I had a weird moment, meeting a lot of new people in my job and everything. It's weird, but it seems like everyone around me still has some semblance of contact with friends from high school, and I don't. I know that plenty of people don't keep close ties with high school friends. I had a little episode this summer when I was home. I was really busy working and going to school. I tried really hard to get in touch with the one friend I still feel positive about. I feel really bad, because I don't really get in touch with people. In high school I took on some friends who ... I don't want to say saved ... because that has a lot of religious implications, but aid in some way or another because I couldn't help my father. After so many years of trying, one friend's problems kept snowballing. She was in her own bubble, her own world. Very, very different.*

73

Ann: I think of two bubbles bouncing up against one another. NI

Berdie: Yeah.

Ann: I think our time is up. Is it OK if Jerry comes to ask you about this session? I

Berdie: Uh huh.

I am suddenly aware that I need to end the session although I have a thought that Berdie is really moving towards something as I cut her off. I am aware that she needs to meet with Jerry right away since she has a class in less than an hour.

POST-SESSION COMMENT

Later, while listening to the tape of this session, I wondered if Berdie experienced me inside a bubble, unable to connect with her. I was not as active in this session as I had been in previous sessions when I had showed her specific study strategies, assessed her learning styles, and sat with her while she completed time-management exercises. She reported that all of this helped her complete her academic semester successfully and helped her feel more motivated. I think that, in retrospect, I was passive because I was being taped and felt the need to restrain myself from offering the kind of practical advice that had emerged in prior sessions. Giving specific advice and creating time schedules didn't seem very congruent with being a client-centered therapist. Yet, Berdie reported that after those sessions she felt more organized, performed better in her courses, and was able to complete her semester successfully.

THE INTERVIEW (REPORTED BY JERRY)

(There are some preliminary comments after we were introduced. She was eating and commented that she was hypoglycaemic. I wondered if she was taking insulin because she seemed on the verge of an insulin reaction. She said she was OK.)

Jerry: Start any way you want.

Berdie: The main thing that strikes me about her in the sessions I have had with her … I have had a number of other sessions with her …

Jerry: How many? NI

I felt the need to have this information for discussing her involvement in therapy. It is the sort of thing that I might forget about if it didn't naturally come up again. I might ask this sort of question in a therapy session because it sometimes assists me to 'sit in the client's world' better.

Berdie: Six or seven times I saw her last spring and then I went home for summer. Mainly I would say that she is extremely passive when it comes to my impression of her professionally.

She is just sitting there and letting me talk which is fine because I have plenty of things generally to talk about going into the session. I know this is so I can organize my thoughts and direction before going. She doesn't ask a lot of questions. She is certainly not at all prying [Berdie considers prying to be distracting.] *I don't feel that she collaborates or adds a whole lot of analysis to my situation that would be nice.*

Jerry: It would be helpful? NI

Berdie: To get someone's outside perspective. Even to the extent of being a little bit critical, not to have someone pass judgment on me, but have someone's outside opinion and saying this is why you are doing that.

Jerry: So you could bounce it off outside

Berdie: Yeah.

Jerry: For example?

Berdie: Mostly we talked about my habits ... related to academics. She has been extremely helpful with that in the past, with conditions of time-management, and she did offer a lot of direction. But it would have been nice if she even asked, 'Why did you do this?' or 'How far back does it go?' And then depending on my answer say ... 'Huh. This is why you do this'. It could be any number of reasons to give me an outside perspective, plant a couple of seeds and make me go home and think more about why I do things, not just that I do them because I am a big believer in getting to the root of the problem and treating the problem.

Jerry: A problem solver?

Berdie: Yeah. [She continues with discussion of how she doesn't get things done until she has to get them done at the last minute ... She mentions never completing a book.]

Jerry: I hardly ever complete a book after I reach the half way mark. I might go back to it. I don't have a lot of discipline to stay on some tasks when my interest wanes ... which is my problem. Essentially if I have a deadline, I get it done. I don't know why that occurs to me. NI

I felt mixed up here. I was thinking that I might not be focused enough on my task of finding out her experience with the therapist, and then felt that I was not communicating what I experienced from 'her view'. So I was thinking that my experience of needing a deadline was similar to her experience and then I wondered why I said anything at all and felt inclined to tell her that I didn't know why this occurred to me.

Berdie: I would say that she is extremely positive and very, very encouraging.

Jerry: So you are kind of getting like [Sound was lost on tape. I was summarizing her way of doing her assignments and coping with her problems] *you feel comfortable and can get it done yourself ... You have had other counselors do it that way and didn't find it helpful.* [Sound on tape lost. I believe that she was referring to therapists helping her to discover why she behaves in certain ways. I was trying to clarify whether or not this is what she meant.] NI

This comment seemed to immediately interfere with discourse. I remember feeling relieved that she did not seem affected by my meandering toward my own 'lack of discipline' in my comment prior to this one. However, I felt that I was pretty much on the mark with my summation of her comments although I don't remember the nature of the discourse at this particular point and could not check it because the sound-track was muffled.

Berdie: Yeah. [Silence for five minutes. She seemed thoughtful.]

Jerry: Have you ... Do you have a specific thing you wished you had talked about or had her ask about?

I decided to break the silence because of my concern that I was not keeping to my task of finding out about her experience with Ann. Normally, if it were a therapy session, I would have most likely waited.

Berdie: Mainly about why I have issues following through. Basically, that is something that permeates every aspect of my life, but it comes to the biggest nastiest head in my academic career. What am I going to practice or not. I used to be really good at science and maths but once I got into it it was too much for me. Science is not my forte. I read and write a lot outside of school. That is actually my strong talent. I am a science major, and I am really bad at maths. I am much more of an English/Philosophy kind of person and every English based course, like anthropology, I take, I ace, but that's just not what I want to be in school for. I have to kick my butt to make it through and every day is a struggle.

Jerry: Now if I were to ask you, 'Why is that?' Is that the kind of question you might want Ann to ask? I

I felt torn between whether to stay with her struggling or to return to my inquiry about her experience with Ann.

Berdie: Basically, I don't feel like we get to a deeper level with most things. What I want to get from a counseling session is anything ... is something I couldn't get on my own. I can sit and write in a journal, which I do a lot. Just to get things out and I'm not ... It's nice to get a nourishing, positive feedback environment. It's good to get it out in that kind of environment and get a little encouragement to do the right thing. But I want to get something I wouldn't get basically having a counseling session with myself. I feel like a lot of times that isn't really there. I know she doesn't want to come across as harsher, judgmental in any way but I don't think it would be too difficult for her at all, or detrimental, to say 'I think this might be why you ...' or even just asking me 'why do you do that?' Or where do you think that comes from? And I'm not a person for psychoanalysis. Well, I am when it comes to myself ... I am way too harsh and judgmental, my thoughts and actions. If it was a positive thing, it could be a good thing as long as it just doesn't bring your self down unnecessarily. [Silence for a minute with a couple of minutes and some comments that are not clear.]

She seems light and happy during this silence somewhat contrary to the mesh of talking about Ann and about herself. She then refers to her view of Ann. She mentions Ann as being able to reach into a bag to give her something. This triggers laughter in me because of things that Ann and I talked about; i.e. Ann's perception of having a Barney Bag in order for her to give something to a client who keeps asking for something 'concrete'.

Jerry: [I muttered something like]: *'I guess she has a bag full of things' and laughed.* NI

This interaction seemed strange in the verbal context but natural in our relationship.

Berdie: That's the only thing I would say. I certainly appreciate the fact that she doesn't try to unnecessarily push me towards anything. That's … There are enough people who do that … even if my therapist didn't prescribe I would have him really, really pressure me a couple of times to see a doctor to prescribe drugs. I saw a guy in the mental health center who did this. I am totally a candidate for ADD medication but I will do anything I can to avoid medication, synthetic medication, over the counter medication, especially with all my blood sugar issues. The fact that pharmaceuticals work differently it's difficult … at least for me. I'm not saying that people don't need it. There are enough of other things I can do … That is an absolute last resort.

Jerry: What you have experienced is that some people have kind of pushed that … [Berdie interrupts.]

Berdie: I have had periods where I was extremely depressed and had doctors prescribe and it worked. I feel like I would really listen to her if she did suggest something like that, because she would be doing the right thing if she would feel that it had got to that point, because a lot of times I can be very excited and stick to my guns a little bit more than I should when it comes to certain things—which is one reason why I basically drove myself to all the health problems that I have right now, by being vegetarian for three years despite my body very, very needing … I think my choices, my emotions, my morals could be the same way. I can stick to my ethical stance over …

Jerry: [Mumbled.]

I feel somewhat caught between staying with her tendency to explore herself and my need to obtain more information about her experience of the therapy session. I realize that she is giving me this information as well and am aware of my anxiety about getting all I can about her session with Ann. I just decide to be quiet.

Berdie: I know once someone says something to me and plants that seed, even if it's still in your head and even if it is completely irrational, it's still in your head and it might not otherwise have been there, so I don't know … I think there's a lot of power in that. [Silence of four minutes. She seems to be reflecting on her statement …]

Berdie: But overall I think she's one of the best I have seen.

Jerry: As you … are you sitting there sometimes in the session with Ann thinking … why doesn't she ask …

I was feeling the ending of the session was approaching and I wanted to be sure that I understood her experience of several specific things about the therapy sessions.

Berdie: Yes and like I said I can't really say ... I want her to take me outside or suggest something.

Jerry: You would like to look at yourself. You would like more to look at yourself some from the outside as well as the inside when you do too much with the inside. NI

Berdie: Well, it is just difficult. It's difficult to focus on something when I am too close to it because you, your situation, your person, yourself won't have you ... I am definitely much better at being an outside observer than being ...

Jerry: So you could be a scientist with yourself?

I thought that I caught it in a nutshell in a way that fitted her view of herself.

Berdie: Yeah.

Jerry: Your recent session with Ann just now. I was wondering about that.

Berdie: Yeah, I thought mostly she just was listening, which helps and is one of her steps, and encouraging and suggesting a little bit of ... I would say something or talk a good while and she would provide a synopsis, but I don't think that she really added that much of her own reflection or suggestion like she did with my time-management, which was extremely helpful in other sessions. Possibly she could even relate to her own experiences and by relating to similar experience but not ... I could say I can see the choices she made in a similar situation and I could learn from those.

Jerry: I ... if you could jump outside of yourself and not be so entangled, so to speak, it's almost like you work so hard inside ... You want to jump outside. NI

Berdie: [Indicates agreement with my statement but sound is lost. Silence. This silence lasted about five minutes.]

Again, I broke it because of my anxiety about the session ending before I covered more of Berdie's experience with Ann.

Jerry: So did Ann ever talk too much?

Berdie: No. I definitely did eighty percent of the talking.

I wanted to be sure to hear Berdie's version of this since Ann had indicated that she feels that she talks too much and, in social discourse, I have found Ann to be talkative. I feel the need to explain this to Berdie.

Jerry: I say this because she kind of sees herself as very talkative. She probably sees herself as very talkative. I

Berdie: Well, from my experiences, depending on what kind of talker you are, a lot of people that can talk well are actually very good listeners depending on their personality.

Jerry: You perceive Ann ... You don't especially want Ann to talk a lot ?

I was puzzled here about understanding Berdie's wish for Ann to be more active and guiding.

Berdie: Not necessarily more, but a little more focused. [Silence of three minutes. She seemed to be very deep in thought.]

Berdie: My main job is being a student. I can get more resolve on this. [Birdie goes on to talk about her parents and complex issues related to their divorce.]

Again, I felt in somewhat of a dilemma here because I think that Berdie was entering one core theme that pervades her struggles and I was pulled by the need to focus on her relationship with Ann.

Jerry: So in terms of your interactions with Ann ... NI

Berdie: Because we have talked about it, it is something I have to field on my own. I'm not using school to get away from anything. Undergraduate is a hurdle getting distance from family issues. Basically, what I am looking for now is personal organization and figuring out how to make myself more productive with no agenda.

Jerry: It sounds like you see Ann as pretty easy to talk with. I

I continue to feel divided between staying with Berdie's direction and focusing on her experiences with Ann.

Berdie: Definitely.

Jerry: It's more related to the outside thing. If I can look at myself then have someone give me something from the outside, I can take it or leave it. NI

Berdie: Yeah, it does help that she is really easy to talk to. [Sound lost.] *I feel right now in that sense I do need, basically, someone to push me about medical issues because when you feel really sick all the time ... and then I feel depressed because I'm not doing much, then I'm not productive. It's a vicious cycle. I feel better when I am productive. I need someone to break it down into little steps and say 'you need to go to the store and buy something for breakfast', 'you need to make an appointment and go see a nutritionist ... see this doctor and that doctor and spend twenty minutes' ... just breaking things down into manageable steps so you have everything planned out for the next month to get yourself in a better place—but if someone can't convince you to do it, ultimately then its useless.*

Jerry: Kind of thinking ... you can do that but you just can't get out of that cycle. NI

Berdie: Not just 'this is what you need to do this' but 'this is why you need to do it' and convince me, tell me a story about (how it will be) one year from now. I need someone to push me. I have massive food allergies. [She goes on to talk about her allergies (i.e. soy), starving herself because she was not eating enough protein.] *I was destructive to myself and my loved ones ... another one of these situations where my morals were overriding my better judgment and I just needed a lot of people, professional people that I respected, to say 'this is what you need to do' and 'this is why you need to do it' and now it's just a matter of constantly keeping up with my body.*

Jerry: That's kind of an example of what you want from Ann? I

79

I try to connect her frame to her experience with Ann, somewhat reluctantly because I experience her chipping away at her clarification of some important things for her.

Berdie: Yeah, motivation, to make a connection in order to fully get all of the motivation.

I wasn't sure that I understood her response, but I was struck by the totality of the things that she viewed as burdening her, and the word 'motivation' stuck with me.

Jerry: You mention depression, ADD, and physical and nutritional problems. These are all kind of on top of you? NI

I felt compelled to check my understanding of what she was saying here.

Berdie: Oh yeah! In a sense they are all easier problems to deal with than situational. Outside influence … decide how you feel about them and handle them—like my father and family—the only thing that will change is how I decide to handle it, which I have lots of years of experience dealing with. With health problems … a lot of vicious cycles. The main thing especially when the blood sugar is low and capacity for action is out the window sometimes …

I am very aware that she continually returns to her conflict within her family and the specific conflict with her father and her references to how she might decide to handle it.

Jerry: [I mention something about situational and internal/health problems being a burden.] *Any special thoughts about Ann. Wondering anything about her?*

Again, I am aware that our session is about over. In fact, the tape ends as I am saying that our time is about up. Berdie talks for another ten minutes about her attempts to gain weight. I thought about a time when several friends and I were in training for athletic events and we had trouble maintaining weight.

Jerry: [I mentioned briefly the time when I had trouble maintaining weight.] *We used to drink double milk shakes with a couple of raw eggs two or three times a day.*

I felt hesitant about saying this to her, thinking that it really had no relevance, but then thought … what if it happened to be a thing that could help her get out of the weight loss problem. It just popped out as I was wondering if I should mention this as we ended the session.

Berdie: UGGH!! My mother used to make me milk shakes to help me …

'That'll teach me,' I thought as we discontinued the interview. I offered my appreciation for her volunteering for the interview. She indicated that she enjoyed talking with me, and we walked across campus together as she directed me toward the bus stop, squeezing each other's hand as we departed.

POST-INTERVIEW COMMENTS

Most of my comments within the session came from recall after reviewing the typescripts. I did not have most of the thoughts during the session or, if I did, they were at a subconscious level of awareness. In retrospect, several things struck me that took place outside of the dialogue.

First, Berdie mentioned briefly during one of the tape sound problems something about the mental health counselor who referred her. She mentioned his family and some things about them. One of my strongest feelings was that of her sadness and regret at not having the kind of family life that she perceived them to be living.

Second, I thought about my remark about a milkshake that I considered to be an inappropriate comment. In retrospect, it might have been meaningful that Berdie felt so free to naturally respond with disdain to the idea. Maybe I stumbled into giving her indirect advice that she often sought and that my statement allowed her to expressively reject it?

Third, Berdie seemed to delight in directing me through the campus to the bus stop and appreciative of our walk together across the campus. Our ending hand-squeeze seemed meaningful to me.

All of these experiences would have been embedded in me if I were to see her as her therapist in the future. I am not sure if, or where, or how, they would fit into the relationship. They might turn out to be irrelevant to her at any given time. They would, however, probably exist as part of my experiencing of her world.

CONCLUSIONS

The intention of this experiment was to examine the client's experience of her therapist and the therapist's experience of the session in order to identify features of a positive psychology. Positive psychology, as noted elsewhere in this book, focuses on well-being, joy, and what makes life worth living, as well as on the elimination of distress, anxiety, and problems. We view positive psychology as existing when the individual:

- experiences fewer *conditions* of positive regard (ultimately experiencing unconditional positive self-regard),
- lives in terms of integration of feelings and self, and
- lives at a higher level of psychological adjustment.

THEORETICAL ASSUMPTIONS

Our functional stance is that of client-centered therapy (Rogers, 1959), wherein our intent is to experience unconditional positive regard toward the client and to experience empathic understanding of the client. We trust that a person will move toward constructive directions if we can maintain our attention to the client's frame of reference and receive the client without judgment. In our vernacular, we strive to relate to the client with *unconditional empathic reception*. In short, we posit that the client will live a more positive life if she is allowed to go in her own direction, at her own pace, and in her own way.

BERDIE AS A CLIENT

The client in this session, Berdie, was able to proceed in her own direction without being interrupted, and felt empowered to continue in her own direction even when therapist responses might have re-directed her. There is some evidence that Berdie benefited from initial counseling sessions. Berdie indicated that early sessions were quite valuable to her. She mentioned that the meetings with Ann saved her. She was able to use time-management and readjust her schedule in a way that allowed her to meet all of her academic and personal obligations and stay in school. She valued the 'Barney Bag' activities (time-management and determining ways to negotiate with her instructors), while also noting that Ann understood her, 'listened well', and that Berdie felt able to talk eighty percent of the time with Ann. Behavioral indices such as elevated grades, increased attendance and decreased anxiety confirmed Berdie's perceptions of gain.

We do not know about positive outcome from this last session with Ann.

Berdie expressed to Ann and Jerry that she would like to have more of Ann's view about what might be helpful. She felt that such expertise might be helpful as long she could reject such suggestions. However, Ann and Jerry offered few suggestions.

THERAPIST AND INTERVIEWER

Our struggles with meeting expectations, other than those that focused on the client's frame of reference, led us to examine the client's responses in an unusual way. Responses were *not* examined with speculations of what responses or actions might have been helpful or what might have been accurate according to usual criteria. We did not have predetermined ideas that Berdie should go through a certain process, nor assumptions that any particular response repertoire was required to understand her frame of reference. Instead, responses were examined by identifying whether or not any given therapist response altered the client's directional process. Did the responses distract the client from the direction of her discourse? How free was the client to pursue her own direction, at her own pace, and in her own way?

For the most part, Berdie (as did the other client involved with the supervision but not reported here) continued in her direction even after responses that we thought might interrupt her. These responses were identified as Non-Interruptive (NI) responses. The responses that did influence her were identified as Interruptive (I) responses. However, the interruptive responses influenced her only for a short time. Our experience with Berdie (and the individual not included in this chapter) generated a couple of speculations about the therapy process.

SPECULATIONS ABOUT THE THERAPY PROCESS

First, we conclude that the relationship and the attitude of therapist non-directivity allowed Berdie to go uninterrupted in her own direction, in her own way, and at her own pace. For example, Jerry's periodic comments to focus Berdie on her therapy with Ann were most often met with short statements followed by a return to Berdie's direction. Jerry's meandering into his own reactions in several instances did not redirect Berdie's direction as we initially thought might happen. Interestingly, the direct questions to Berdie about her experience with Ann did not interfere with Berdie's continuation of her own direction. We speculate that the overall receptive attitude of the interviewer as well as the general interest in her frame of reference created this freedom. Likewise, the same phenomena occurred with Berdie in her session with Ann. Berdie perceived Ann as listening at least 'eighty per cent of the time', and as one of the best of several therapists who Berdie had experienced.

Second, Ann did not feel the need to reach into her Barney Bag for practical suggestions or to suggest a book, nor did she offer all of her analogies to Berdie. Ann thought of metaphors that she might have shared, but did not, in this session. These metaphors were Ann's way of understanding part of Berdie's world. The metaphors had no instructive intent. However, the Barney Bag was there, perhaps, for the therapist's security and for concrete activities a client might seek. Both Ann and Jerry had deep trust in the client's way, pace, and direction.

Third, it became more obvious to us that therapists' ways of experiencing another person's world differ. Berdie's interview with Jerry consisted of many of her struggles that were presented in her counseling session with Ann. We have to wonder if Berdie's direction would have been altered for very long if Ann had reached more into her Barney Bag to meet Berdie's wish. We doubt it—as long as the stance remained dedicated to Berdie's frame of reference. We also wonder if Berdie's direction would have been interrupted with an empathic understanding response. Jerry could have, for example, responded to Berdie's several references to her situation with her father (something that came up several times in both sessions and a couple of times in the summarized comments although not verbally noted). For example, Jerry had the thought of saying something like, 'So dealing with your father is no longer a thing that you can do anything about'. This was directly stated by Berdie but might also be considered as something 'on the edge' of further meaning. Such a statement might have encouraged further exploration by Berdie. However, the fact was that Jerry didn't need to ask her anything to check his understanding of her meaning (the only real reason for an empathic response according to Rogers). We have to wonder whether or not such a comment, even if accurate and leading to greater exploration, would have distracted Berdie from *her way* of processing and exploration? If Jerry had responded in this way, he would still trust that Berdie would return to her direction and way. However, such a response would have been no less of an interruption than the somewhat meaningless reference to a milkshake (pulled from Jerry's Barney Bag). It seems that if the receptive attitude and relational involvement is there, and if the therapist doesn't say too much, then what the therapist actually says is not as important as how the therapist is in the relationship with the client. The client goes in her own direction if she views the therapist's presence as accepting, supporting, and in search of her perception of the world, rather than with an intent of directing her.

Most examinations of therapist–client interactions are predicated upon pre-determined directions that the client should go; that is to more feeling, or greater depth, or resolution of problems, or diminished symptoms. Even analyses of client-centered therapy sessions have been viewed from the perspective of asking what kind of verbal responses encourage the client's self-development and self-direction. Our discovery with Berdie suggests that, quite simply, the receptive stance allows clients the freedom to go in their own direction and, in fact, to assert themselves to go in that direction. Berdie's direction was more determined by the lack of interference, perhaps enabled in part by the very presence of Ann with her Barney Bag as a security for her receptive stance to Berdie's world.

Contrary to conventional thought, facilitative responses are those that do not interfere with the client's direction rather than those that encourage clarification. It is the freedom created for the client to go in her own direction, at her own pace and in her own way. The tendency of the client is to direct herself when free to do so.

We wonder if Jerry's strong experience of Berdie's silent longing for a 'loving family', her spontaneous reaction to Jerry's 'unhelpful' milk shake comment, her post-session guidance to Jerry to find the bus stop and the hand-squeezing departure with Jerry revealed a positive constructive development.

In her counseling session with Ann, Berdie is able to articulate precisely what she needs. She needs someone to 'push' her and 'convince' her to do the things she feels that she needs to do. She wants more personal organization to break a vicious cycle of being ill and procrastinating so that she can be free and more productive. Ann's lack of presuppositions about the way the counseling session would unfold, her willingness to try to understand Berdie's world, and her belief and trust in Berdie being able to find her own self-directive variables did not interfere with Berdie's ability to articulate what it is that she needs. Just as Berdie was able to articulate to Ann precisely what she needs, she was equally articulate with Jerry about what she needs in counseling from Ann. Our experience with Berdie (and the other client not reported here) suggests that it is the non-judgmental, unconditional, receptive relationship of non-interference that frees the client to activate her innate constructive direction. The Barney Bag represents access to maximal personal participation in the relationship while remaining dedicated to unconditional empathic reception of the person.

REFERENCES

Bozarth, JD (1998) *Person-Centered Therapy: A revolutionary paradigm.* Ross-on-Wye: PCCS Books.

Bozarth, JD (2002) The Specificity Myth: The Fallacious Premise of Mental Health Treatment. Paper presentation at the American Psychological Association Convention. <http://personcentered.com/specificity.htm> 10/01/07.

Glazer, T and Grean, C (1994) *Barney Live* [Video]. The United States: Songs Music and Grean Music.

Lambert, M (1992) Psychotherapy outcome research. In JC Norcross and MR Goldfried (eds) *Handbook of Psychotherapy Integration* (pp. 94–129). New York: Basic Books.

Rogers, CR (1957) The necessary and sufficient conditions of therapeutic personality change. *Journal of Consulting Psychology, 21*, 95–103.

Rogers, CR (1959) A theory of therapy, personality, and interpersonal relationships as developed in the client-centered framework. In S Koch (ed) *Psychology: A Study of a Science, Vol. 3: Formulations of the person and the social context* (pp. 184–256). New York: McGraw-Hill.

CHAPTER 8

RECOVERING FROM CHILDHOOD SEXUAL ABUSE: DISSOCIATIVE PROCESSING

JAN HAWKINS

And you O my soul where you stand,
Surrounded, detached, in measureless oceans of space,
Ceaselessly musing, venturing, throwing, seeking the spheres to connect them,
Till the bridge you will need be form'd, till the ductile anchor hold,
Till the gossamer thread you fling catch somewhere, O my soul

(Whitman, 1855)

Childhood sexual abuse can have long-term effects on those who survive it (Hawkins, 2005). For some, the trauma leads to the development of different selves, each split and separate from the other, each holding their own memories, skills and realities. For those children who survived the overwhelming psychic confusion and pain of betrayal by those they thought loved them by leaving their body, numbing physically, depersonalising or otherwise defending themselves psychically, there can be long-term problems. For whilst this creative defence mechanism of dissociation protects from the full realisation of what is happening, it can later prevent healing and cause difficulties in relationships. Having learned to dissociate to survive, that very dissociation can block a healthy integrated development as the child grows to adulthood. In this chapter I discuss Sarah, who suffered repeated sexual abuse as a child by a close relation and survived by dissociating from the pain and confusion. Though many clients who experience this degree of distress feel they are mad and many are indeed labelled and diagnosed with frightening (yet vague) mental illnesses when they seek help for the symptoms that only hint at their suffering, dissociation is actually a chimerical survival strategy. Dissociation, otherwise known as 'double consciousness', is a normal aspect of everyday living for all people. It is most often seen in the phenomenon, familiar to most, of travelling from A to B without any clear memory of having made the various steps of that journey because the mind was otherwise occupied. Double consciousness allows us to drive a car whilst carrying on a conversation. Dissociation is double consciousness in the extreme, allowing the person to live through a considerably painful ordeal whilst floating on the ceiling watching it happen to a different person. Sarah's dissociation meant that she was not able to understand or manage her distressing symptoms until she met the 'others' in her and was finally able to acknowledge the harm she had suffered as a child.

THE CLIENT'S PRESENTING ISSUES

Sarah's first contact with me was on the telephone, where she checked out whether I had any understanding of the experience of abuse. I was struck by the clarity of purpose and felt almost interviewed. This impressed me, and I must have passed the interview because she came to see me wearing a business suit and carrying a leather-bound folder of writing, which she mentioned but did not share in that first session. Sarah swiftly laid out the issues she wanted to work on: her history of abuse, an eating disorder and vague allusions to self-harming behaviours, fears about her own anger, confusion about her sexual identity. She described difficulties with rigid thinking and classifying and then confusion when things didn't fit. She told me, too, that she cast men in her life in the role of brother but then sexualised the relationships. Despite this, she was living with her partner, a woman whom she had met at a youth club when she was just fifteen. At the time Sarah had had a crush on the youth worker who had, one day, kissed her passionately. This led very quickly to Sarah moving in with the woman and they had subsequently lived together for ten years. Sarah felt guilty about this relationship, particularly because of her different relationships with men during this time. She wanted to leave the relationship but felt she would be letting her partner down. She was very confused about her sexuality, feeling she had to meet her partner's sexual needs even though she had to 'numb out' whilst doing so.

My impression after this very full session was that Sarah was very much a high flier and on the brink of collapse. She had managed to live with the legacy of her childhood abuse, in part with the diversion of her success in her career as a high achieving architect. In part she had managed to live with the long-term effects of abuse by being capable of hiding her eating disorder and other difficulties. These had begun to catch up with her and she had decided she needed to work in therapy on these issues. As I came to know her I realised that she was approaching therapy with the same drive and determination as she had approached other things in her life. I have rarely counselled anyone who worked so hard and so fast at her healing. I know there were several occasions when I felt I just had to encourage her to be gentle with herself and to acknowledge the drivenness of her desire to 'get better'.

THE RELATIONSHIP WITH THE CLIENT

After that first session, I reflected that a rapport had quickly been established. Sarah was someone who was open to relationship and was clear about what she needed in a therapist: someone who could listen to what had happened to her and help her. My sense was that the 'help' she needed was to be accepted as the high flying, driven person she was but, at the same time, I realised that I must not be overwhelmed by the speed of her thinking and talking. My sense was that there was little Sarah needed from me; she seemed so informed and sophisticated in describing what she needed to work on. However, I had a sense that this fast talking, energised woman needed me to be aware of a vulnerability very close to the surface. I did not perceive any incongruity in Sarah, rather my sense was that there may be more to her than was immediately present. This was a feeling in me, with nothing tangible to go on, and I recognised that I would need to be careful not to make assumptions, or try to 'connect the dots'. Psychological contact was established very quickly and was maintained throughout our work together; though it soon became clear that there was more than one 'Sarah' and that whilst psychological contact was always present, it was with different selves at different times. Sometime this meant that I was the facilitator between discrete selves.

For some survivors of childhood abuse, the only way to survive the overwhelming confusion and physical pain of what is happening is to dissociate. Dissociation is the psyche's ingenious survival strategy which spontaneously divides the consciousness so that the individual may describe not being present, or disintegrating, or watching from the ceiling when the abuse was taking place. Sometimes the trauma is so intense that the experience is of a freezing in time and another child seems to appear to continue living when the abused child cannot go on. Often the child who appears is highly adapted, having learned what is necessary to be accepted. Sarah became a very high achiever but that was only one aspect of her developing self. She did very well at school, learned languages quickly and spoke them fluently, and to the outer world she seemed to be independent and popular. Like many survivors of abuse who survive by diverting all their energies into achieving, the cost is often intense isolation when feelings of depression arise. Sarah was sometimes brought to the brink of collapse either by sudden severe feelings of despair or by feelings of rage with violent images. She could not work out why this happened, and this lack of ability to understand what was happening for her challenged her self concept as one who was incredibly bright.

In our first few sessions, Sarah brought, and would read to me, long, intense and incredibly sophisticated poetry. I would sometimes struggle to understand some of the words or to grasp the imagery. Yet there was an emotional quality to them all that I could connect with. It seemed essential to Sarah, in these first sessions, to relate her difficulties in the form of poetry. Whilst she could seem relaxed and engaged in the earliest stages of each session (and as we came to the end of each) for talking about what she was feeling and struggling with, she needed to read her poetry. I stayed with this and attempted to express my understanding of the emotional undercurrents expressed within all the words and form of poetry. After some weeks, I gently invited her to explore how the poetry was working for her and it was during that exploration that our relationship shifted gear. From then until the end of our work together things took an entirely different path and she rarely spoke through her written poetry again.

PROGRESS, SESSION BY SESSION

In our first session the warmth and rapport was great. I liked Sarah instantly. She had talked about working with a therapist before who she acknowledged she had protected from the abuse. She had felt that the therapist was not able to deal with her abuse issues.

She had, she said, tried to talk about it but could see he was uncomfortable and then had avoided talking about it. I wondered how much of this discomfort was Sarah's in discussing the issues at all. Perhaps, too, there may have been some discomfort in her discussing the issues with a man. Or perhaps the therapist had not explored fully enough what his own feelings, attitudes and beliefs were in relation to childhood sexual abuse. My concern, however, was to convey my own willingness and openness to explore whatever Sarah needed to explore. I had stated firmly that I hoped she wouldn't feel she had to protect me from it. This was when she read her first poem to me.

As the subsequent sessions developed, the poetry conveyed her confusion, anger and fast-paced lifestyle. Running away from what was hurting inside, trust was deepening. It was then that Sarah began to express her fear of the degree of trust she was feeling in me. This exploration initially came in the form of a poem whose meaning was obscured behind many words, metaphors and images. I felt that I had cracked the code and she was clearly relieved that I had understood this fear of trust. She was then able to explore this further, wondering why she had felt this trust from the beginning with me and saying she felt she had somehow always known me. Strangely enough, that feeling was present for me too. Despite the fear of this trust Sarah continued to place her trust in me.

It was during a session where she had decided to try to speak her truth without the poems that her usual fast-paced, sophisticated delivery stopped abruptly and suddenly she moved from the chair she was sitting in to the floor, where she adopted a cross-legged position. Her whole posture and demeanour changed. Her face changed completely and when she spoke it was with an entirely different voice. This was only the second time in my work as a therapist that I had encountered such a sudden change of person and I was momentarily stunned. Quickly though, I was engaged with a small child, an impish, mischievous little girl called Susie, who giggled a lot and smiled widely and talked about Sarah. She laughed conspiratorially when telling me that she liked chocolate but that Sarah didn't like chocolate. Susie had eaten 'lots and lots of chocolate and made Sarah be sick'. Susie told me she saw a lot of what Sarah did and how Sarah pretended to be clever but wasn't really. She told me that she didn't mind being sick but Sarah hated it. Sarah thought she would die when she was sick but Susie was never going to die. I asked Susie how old she was and learned that she was six years old. She was delightful! Every now and then she would play with her hair and ask 'do you think my hair is pretty?' or 'do you like my party dress?' touching what was obviously, to her, a dress she was wearing. In fact she was in her usual business trouser suit.

As the session was nearing an end I felt the need to ensure that Sarah was able to come back to herself—it felt irresponsible to send a six-year-old out into the street alone! I asked Susie where Sarah was, and suddenly Sarah was back—back in her chair and slightly dazed. I asked if she was aware of what had happened and it appeared that she had been absent for the time when Susie was talking. As the end of the session was so close I decided to focus on how she was in that moment and made our next appointment. At this point she was completely back to the Sarah I knew.

This session was a turning point. I realised now that I had two clients rather than one and I needed to be very careful for the next few sessions to remember who had told me what. Susie seem to know all about Sarah and enjoyed telling me tales about what Sarah had been doing, especially if she had been clumsy or done things that made Susie laugh. Sarah, on the other hand, did not seem to be aware of Susie at all.

It became clear to me that part of the effect of Sarah's early sexual abuse was development of discrete selves. This experience is often pathologised in the psychiatric tradition and has been variously described as multiple personality disorder (MPD), then as manipulation and fantasy (i.e. not real at all) and currently is recognised as dissociative identity disorder (DID). Because of the word 'disorder' it can be very frightening for the individual who experiences themselves as multiple selves. Quite apart from any confusion due to the conflicts of needs, views, memories, abilities and so on of the different individuals, there is a fear of judgement by others. I prefer the term 'different selves' as this describes what individuals experience—and does not judge. In psychiatric terms, the aim of 'treatment' is to integrate the different selves, or at least to bring the selves into harmony. For those interested, the film of the book *Sybil* (Schreiber, 1973) gives a clear example of the causes and experiences of living with different selves. Unfortunately, the end of the film is given Hollywood treatment implying that it is possible to bring all the selves together in one dramatic and loving session. The truth is far more complicated of course, though the film does show how quickly personalities may interchange, and therefore how much is needed from the therapist. The experience of recognising different selves can be terrifying, repeating the isolation and fear that was present at the time of the abuse which caused the fragmentation of the self. This experience is expressed by Dr Cameron West in his moving *First Person Plural* (1999).

I was present with Sarah when Susie emerged. I quickly realised what a privileged position I was in and how important it was for me to hold Susie's presence as separate from Sarah's until Sarah came to a point of awareness herself. As a person-centred practitioner, it is important to stay with my client's awareness and not to bring my own into the space. To do so risks jolting my client's process and taking control of the pace of the work. For those unfamiliar with the dissociative experience it can be shocking as well as frightening to witness a client shift so dramatically. There is a double-edged danger, for those who have not encountered such clear evidence of trauma, to either pathologise the client, possibly considering them psychotic, or even to be fabricating their experience. The other danger is of feeling a need to 'rescue' the client from the dissociative state in order to regain a sense of control or competence. There are times with some clients, who share different selves in the way Sarah did, that I discuss with my client the possibility of creating a wider time-boundary for our sessions, to allow for safe processing of the most distressing material which may provoke dissociation. The 'therapeutic hour' is not always an adequate container for some clients. I find that sessions of one and a half hours or two hours work better for certain clients when they are in the most intense phase of their healing from childhood abuse. Keeping the discussion about timing collaborative allows for individual need, as well as sharing of the power in our relationship. Sarah though, seemed to have an inner rhythm which allowed us always to be on safe ground as each session finished. Until I was confident of this, and having met

Susie for the first time, I always arranged Sarah's session as the last of that day to allow for recovery time if that were needed. Conveying a sense of trust in the client to regain the adult functioning, more grounded sense of self, in my experience, ensures that the client is empowered. On those rare occasions with other clients who have needed that recovery time, a period of time quietly alone in the therapy room whilst I make tea and bring them back to the business of what they will do next, has always resulted in the client being safe to leave.

Then came a session where I sensed that Sarah had a vague connection to what had been happening in her absence. Her shift back to herself from Susie had left her disoriented and with a vague feeling of having been 'somewhere else'. She asked, in her usual businesslike fashion, for some feedback. It was then that I mentioned having met Susie. This disclosure prompted Sarah into telling me she did know about Susie but had always felt too embarrassed to tell anyone. She asked what Susie had been saying. I recall momentarily wondering about confidentiality for Susie but that thought flashed in and out of my mind. Susie, it seemed, had always lived on the edge of Sarah's awareness, but Sarah had not been able to hear what she was saying. I can only imagine that this was because when Susie appeared, Sarah disappeared.

Susie was completely unharmed by the abuse. She talked about the relative who had abused Sarah. She was happy about him and laughed when talking about the fun they had. It seems Susie was oblivious of any of the sexual abuse. She was simply happy, engaging and rather precocious. She seemed to be aware that Sarah didn't know what she had been saying while she knew all about Sarah and thought that very funny. It was Susie who introduced me to Wendy. When Wendy appeared, again Sarah's whole demeanour, posture and voice changed. She seemed very, very young and thought of Susie as her protector. Wendy did not talk about Sarah but about being very frightened when Susie would make people look at them because she would dance or sing. I had already noticed how my body language and voice changed when I was with Susie and it changed again with Wendy. I found that I was responding exactly as if the person in front of me was three (Wendy) or six (Susie). When I was speaking with Sarah I was speaking with an adult with an adult's vocabulary. Wendy had a far more limited vocabulary than Susie. She was much more timid and talked about wanting to hide but Susie not letting her. When Sarah had allowed herself to put down her prepared poetry and talk from herself, the 'others' of her had been able to break through. Susie occasionally complained that Sarah had kept them all up all night and that she was tired and wanted me to tell Sarah off for this. Susie liked staying up late, she'd said, but not when she was too tired!

The process changed again when Sarah began to talk more about the sexual abuse she had experienced. Sometimes Susie would intervene and just want to talk about games she liked playing or tell jokes. I understood that Susie was protecting Sarah when the feelings became too intense. Over time Sarah came to understand this and began to make time to play rather than working the extremely long hours she had been used to. Susie and Wendy were very happy about this. Connections were being made between them and Sarah was beginning to make links between her sexual abuse and the relationship she was living in. A period of intense pain and regret followed as she became overwhelmed with guilt feelings as she recognised that she really did not want to continue the relationship with her long-term partner. Susie had told me about a man Sarah 'loved' in the singsong teasing manner children reveal such things. Sarah was struggling with her feelings about this attraction and the loyalty she felt towards her partner.

We engaged in exploration about Sarah's sexual identity. During this period, neither Susie nor Wendy appeared. Sarah wondered if her sexual abuse had 'made' her a lesbian. She was confused as to whether she was, in fact, a lesbian and confused about sexual feelings generally. At this point, it felt as if direct answers to direct questions were appropriate. It is easy for adults, sexually abused as children, to wonder if it is this that has 'caused' their sexual orientation. It is also part of the pathologising and homophobic culture within psychiatry to assume that abuse does cause the person to become gay or lesbian. However, if it were true that women abused as children by men would become lesbian as a reaction against men, then the proportion of women survivors who are lesbians would be much greater. Similarly, if men abused by women as boys became gay as a reaction against women, there would be far more gay male survivors. If women sexually abused as children by women and boys sexually abused as children by men became gay as a result, there would be strikingly more gay and lesbian women and men than there are in the general population. This is not the case. Interestingly, there seems to be little discussion of the possibility that women and men abused as children who are heterosexual are so as a result of their abuse, either as a reaction against the gender of their abuser or as learned behaviour towards their own gender.

Sexual orientation is about the person's authentic self. Like all other conditions of worth, sexual abuse conditions the child to do what is necessary to gain the approval of the adult or to at least keep safe from further harm. The more conditions of worth there are, the further away from the authentic self the person is. It is only within the authentic self that sexual orientation is truly discernable. What happens with abuse is that the child is engaged in sexual behaviours, and sexual behaviours can happen with anyone irrespective of sexual orientation. For Sarah, her sexual orientation was not a part of her consciousness at the time that she developed her crush on her youth worker. She was a high achieving adolescent whose memories of her own sexual abuse were known but tightly contained within her. She described herself as a 'late developer' in that her friends were all involved with boyfriends and she had not really got any interests outside of her studies—but she did really like her youth worker. This youth worker clearly developed great affection for Sarah, and Sarah craved affection. During our work she realised that her abuser had treated her as a 'princess' telling her how special she was. The youth worker communicated similar feelings about her 'uniqueness' and beauty. When the youth worker kissed Sarah, she felt confused. She was excited to be seen as 'grown up' enough for this and also felt it meant she had a special place in the woman's heart. This was very important to her. She relied on the woman, who cared about her in a way she desperately needed. When she invited her to move in with her Sarah did so happily. Their sexual relationship was always difficult for Sarah. In order to engage sexually, she needed to remove herself from her body. She would 'blank out', staring at the ceiling till she felt she was part of the ceiling. She learned what she had to do to please her partner, but always felt uncomfortable and tried to avoid sex. She loved their physical affection and craved that always, and the cost of that was having to engage in sex too. Sometimes, during sex, she would fantasise—always about men. This confused her terribly. She felt disloyal to her partner and didn't understand why she could be doing one thing while thinking of another. Having grown through late adolescence into adulthood within this relationship, Sarah felt she owed her partner much for supporting her through her training to be an architect. A period of much confusion and pain pushed her to her limits. Anger arose when she considered the age difference between them and how vulnerable she had been as a fifteen-year-old when their relationship had begun. She could not bear to be angry with her partner so turned this on herself and began harming herself through bingeing, vomiting, and cutting. As the pain and tension intensified Susie reappeared in our sessions. Susie informed me when Sarah had cut herself and I was able to support Sarah in ensuring that she had sterile blades and dressings available. This implicitly acknowledged that the cutting was, at the time, a way of easing the tension, but also conveyed my care and concern for Sarah.

Survivors of childhood abuse engage in self-harming behaviours as coping strategies. For some, alcohol or other drugs may serve to anaesthetise a pain that is too intense. For those who did not receive sufficient love, acceptance, comfort and soothing as young children, especially when abuse was part of their experience, it is almost impossible to tolerate their own feelings. When the pain or memories overwhelm, then anything that allows the person to distance themselves from it may be employed. Cutting is a particular form of self-harming which can expose the individual to more pathologising. If the person has required hospital treatment for stitching, they can often be treated with considerable contempt. Some report having to endure stitching without local anaesthetic. There is a lack of understanding of the fact that, whilst the self-harming behaviour may have occurred in a dissociated state, the person may have come to themselves in need of stitching and have no dissociation to numb the pain. Some report being left endlessly waiting and being told they don't have the same rights as those whose injuries were not self-inflicted. The majority of people who cut, like Sarah, keep their self-harming a secret. It is now understood that the majority of self-cutting (and other self-harming behaviours) occurs in a dissociated state. The person has become overwhelmed by feelings and/or memories and has numbed, left their body, feels unreal (depersonalised) or has a discrete self who needs to cut. The act of cutting can be experienced as making the self feel again; making the self real again; letting the 'badness' out; putting the inner pain on the outside where it can be 'dealt with'; loss of control over the one who wants to self-harm. Sarah had developed sophisticated ways of cutting herself which could be covered by her business suits—no-one had known. In the main, I learned, even her partner rarely glimpsed the wounds. For Sarah, the drawing of blood brought her back to herself and, though she did not understand why she 'had' to do it, she had come to accept that this was a part of her life that had to be endured. I did not encounter a separate self-harming self in Sarah. Susie simply told me that Sarah did it and when Sarah spoke about it she did so in typical businesslike fashion, as though it were a part of her life that she accepted. The feelings and triggers to cutting herself were different than those associated with her bingeing and vomiting. This latter behaviour made Sarah feel very ashamed.

Throughout this phase of our work Sarah occasionally mentioned her eating disorder and we would spend time exploring it and how she wanted to make changes. Over time she was able to make links between the feelings she had just before a binge and those she had felt when her abuser had forced oral sex on her as a child. Huge anger was released as she acknowledged the harm this had done to her. At this point it was clear that she had been blaming herself for the abuse, as most survivors do. She had been thinking, as the adult she was then, that she should have stopped it. Having reconnected with Susie and Wendy, she realised that such a small child could not have done anything to stop the abuse. She had been powerless. Violent images and nightmares ensued for a period of time and these needed to be explored in our sessions. During this time Susie would sometimes appear and give Sarah some respite. Sometimes Susie and Wendy would alternate. I felt strongly that I must not favour one over the other, but must stay present to whoever was in the room at the time. I was able to ask each where the other was and this was especially important towards the end of sessions when I felt it was essential to have Sarah back and ready to face the world again.

OUTCOME

During the whole time we were working together, Sarah managed to continue with her hectic work schedule seemingly never missing a beat. She told me that Susie had occasionally interrupted her at work but that she had been able to be firm with her and promised her time when she got home. As we rode the storm that was her rage and sadness, another self appeared. This was Peaceful who seemed to be a discrete aspect of the self who was calm, grounded, rooted and carried Sarah's spiritual being. Sarah was so happy to have this Peaceful appear and felt soothed by her whenever she came. Peaceful only spoke to me herself on two occasions. Both were to assure me she was looking after Sarah, Susie and Wendy.

Gradually Sarah was able to call on Peaceful when feelings were threatening to overwhelm her. She made the decision that she needed to leave her partner. And our work turned to an exploration of how she would achieve this without being overwhelmed with guilt or her partner's pleading. She began to consider dreams for her future (something she had never allowed herself to do before). Sarah seemed to have integrated her selves in a way that filled me with awe. There was now a dialogue between them, though I am fairly sure Susie and Wendy were always spared the memory of the sexual abuse which had begun when Sarah was seven years old.

Our work ended when Sarah had left her partner and had begun to explore a relationship with her new friend. She was clear that she would live alone to allow herself to take this relationship at a pace she felt able to manage. She had stopped having violent disturbing nightmares and had been managing a healthy eating plan for some months. She now recognised the triggers that would previously compel her to binge and vomit and she was able to take action to comfort herself. Without us actually spending time focusing on the eating disorder it seemed to have lost its power over her due to dealing with the underlying distress which had now been processed. I will never forget Susie's delightful smile and wave as sometimes—sure as I had been that Sarah was back and ready for the world—I would glimpse Susie waving delightedly.

REFLECTION

Throughout our work together I was intensely aware of the relationships I had with Sarah, Susie, Wendy and, briefly, with Peaceful. Each relationship felt unique though they were also part of the whole relationship I had with Sarah. I felt intuitively that it was essential to show 'multi-directional partiality' (O'Leary, 1999) favouring none over the others. There were times, when Sarah seemed to be facing very difficult feelings, when Susie would take over and the mood, subject and entire situation would suddenly shift. I felt I had to shift too, whilst holding on to where Sarah had been so that I could come back to her without losing her thread. It was within a relationship that the harm was done and it felt essential that there was a relationship where healing could take place. Sarah was acutely aware of what could have been made of her difficulties and had managed to avoid letting her GP know how much she suffered. Aside from her eating disorder and cutting behaviours and the terrible headaches she suffered, she remained a very healthy woman. She had never disclosed any of these problems to her GP as she feared being referred to a psychiatrist. She was convinced that she would be sectioned if she did see a psychiatrist. She had carefully chosen who she would risk disclosing the full extent of her difficulties to. She intuitively sensed that she could heal and that she would need somebody who believed that too. As a person-centred practitioner, I am endeavouring to provide my clients with a blend of the core attitudinal qualities of empathy, congruence and unconditional regard. I reflected in supervision from time to time on how much energy I was expending holding each of Sarah's selves. Yet that energy never seemed draining. I found it easy to love each of them and could tell how much they needed that.

> The therapist's task is thus formidable for he or she has somehow to rekindle hope in the client's heart and that is impossible without the rediscovery of trust ... Psychological skills, therapeutic insights, sophisticated medication may all have their part to play in the process of healing but, as St. Paul put it in another context, without love they are likely in the end to profit nothing. (Thorne, 1998: 108)

Sarah had taken on the conditions of worth of her parents, becoming a high achiever who led a driven and sophisticated life. But her existence was far removed from her deeper organismic self. When Peaceful arrived, I had a sense that she had reconnected to her own process. Peaceful would certainly not have fitted in with parental requirements.

It was essential too that I understood the function and process of dissociation. Without this understanding, I may well have feared that Sarah was becoming psychotic the first time Susie appeared. Survivors of abuse can often be misperceived as having entered psychotic states due to the manifestations of their dissociation. Here, the definition of psychosis is a loss of shared reality. For those unfamiliar with the manifestations of dissociation there may be a tendency to leap to the assumption of psychosis when faced with a client who may be staring, rocking, unresponsive, switching to a childlike voice, posture, habits. These behavioural manifestations are clues to possible dissociative selves. Sarah reported other classic clues to this experience when she was struggling: feeling paralysed, numb, terrified, spacy, floating, confused, distant, disconnected. She reported suffering from blinding headaches when tension was particularly bad and would then find herself engaged in a different activity (often bingeing) without her headache. The indicators of her having dissociated at the time of the abuse came in her reports that 'I left my body and went to the ceiling', 'I knew it was happening but I thought about something else'. Sarah, Susie, Wendy and Peaceful were all real selves.

This type of dissociative experience can be seen along a continuum where, at one end, lie the 'configurations' of Self described by Mearns and Thorne (2000).

> A 'configuration' is a hypothetical construct denoting a coherent pattern of feelings, thoughts and preferred behavioural responses symbolised or pre-symbolised by the person as reflective of a dimension of existence within the Self. (Mearns and Thorne, 2000: 102)

At the other end of the continuum are the multiple selves who are far from being hypothetical constructs but are real discrete individuals who may not be aware of each other's existence. In Sarah's case, Susie and Wendy were known to her but she was unaware of what they were doing or saying at times. When Peaceful appeared it seemed as if Sarah had reconnected with her authentic self. It was Peaceful who mediated between her selves and brought harmony.

Even if I had not feared psychosis, without understanding dissociation I may have passed on my own lostness and anxiety to Sarah, who had quite enough to deal with without having to face that. Because childhood traumatic abuse can often result in dissociative process, and sometimes can lead to the experience of multiple selves as it did for Sarah, it is important that therapists make themselves aware of how dissociation may manifest within their work.

Within the person-centred approach there is an important sense in which diagnostics are irrelevant. We would seek to avoid pathologising a client's difficulties. On the other hand it would be naive and irresponsible to avoid learning something about the particular issues with which our client's may be struggling. By understanding and accepting Sarah's dissociated selves she was more able to accept and embrace them herself. Her fear of going mad abated and she was able to integrate these selves in such a way that she became multi-dimensional rather than the almost one-dimensional fast paced, driven high flier who was not able to talk about herself except through her poetry. Acceptance of her self-harming episodes and eating disorder as evidence of her distress rather than as something 'wrong' with her, allowed her to focus on the distress and these behaviours gradually diminished as she expressed more of her pain and rage about her experiences of abuse. Acceptance too of her sexual identity confusion at the beginning of the therapy allowed Sarah to recognise that her sexual development had been derailed by her abuser and, subsequently, also by the youth worker. Sarah had not had the space in her life to be in touch with her own sexuality because she had been involved in meeting her abuser's sexual needs and later her confusion between her crush on the youth worker and needs for affection, muddled up with sex, had taken her further away from her own sense of her sexual self. During the therapy, Sarah came to be more in touch with her own sexuality, and experienced desire for the first time. She was beginning to reconnect with her 'directional organismic processes' (Rogers, 1963), her true authentic self. It had also been essential that I had been able to accept Sarah's, and especially Susie's, love for her abuser. Despite her rage at him for what he had done, she loved him very much and needed to know that I understood and accepted that. Acceptance of the total reality of the other selves was another important feature of our work. There is a danger in those who do not have the experience themselves of discrete selves, that an assumption is made that these are simply 'aspects' of self or 'sub personalities' (i.e. Rowan, 1989), or in person-centred terms 'configurations' of self (Mearns and Thorne, 2000). Whilst those terms relate to real experiences for many people, for those whose experience is of real separate selves who have different identities, different skills and different memories, it is very painful to find that these selves are not believed or acknowledged.

My experience of loving Sarah, Susie, Wendy and Peaceful developed very early in our relationship. I felt that Sarah could feel that love, and that her love was *received* was equally important. I had a deep respect for Sarah and trusted that each time she left a session, no matter how painful that session had been, she would go on with her life and stay safe. Her self-harming episodes concerned me as evidence of the degree of her distress but she never expressed any suicidal ideation nor gave any evidence of being at risk. Sarah's survival as a powerful, dynamic and highly skilled woman had depended on her creative functional defence in dissociation. Susie had not needed to know about the abuse and could remain innocent, spontaneous, precocious and fun loving. Wendy was shy and timid but she did not have to know about the abuse and could be alongside Susie for security. Sarah had defended herself from conscious awareness of the harm she had suffered by splitting and focusing on her studies. Her need to self-harm, her bingeing and vomiting and sexual confusion were disconnected from her memories of sexual abuse. This disconnection allowed her to function well in her life. 'Peaceful' was her deeper, spiritual core-self who was able to emerge and bring harmony when it was safe enough to fully acknowledge the pain and confusion of the childhood sexual abuse. With her companions Sarah's identity was enriched; she was more fully herself—or her 'selves'.

When we had completed our work together she had overcome her need to self-harm with the help of Peaceful, who became a more prominent companion. There had been no binge/vomit episodes for some time before we ended and she was looking forward to enjoying life before her fast-paced frenzied work schedule. Sarah led her own process of therapy and recovery, along with Susie, Wendy and Peaceful. As a person-centred therapist I seek to accompany rather than lead. Our work left me in awe of Sarah's ability to have survived and of the pace and breadth of her healing from her abuse.

REFERENCES

Hawkins, J (2005) Living with pain: Mental health and the legacy of childhood abuse. In S Joseph and R Worsley (eds) *Person-Centred Psychopathology: A positive psychology of mental health* (pp. 226–42). Ross on Wye: PCCS Books.

Mearns, D and Thorne, B (2000) *Person-Centred Therapy Today: New frontiers in theory and practice.* London: Sage.

O'Leary, CJ (1999) *Counselling Couples and Families: A person-centred approach.* Thousand Oaks, CA: Sage.

Rogers, CR (1963) The actualising tendency in relation to 'motives' and to consciousness. In M Jones (ed) *Nebraska Symposium on Motivation* (pp. 1–24). Lincoln, NE: University of Nebraska Press.

Rowan, J (1989) *Subpersonalities: The people inside us.* London and New York: Routledge.

Schreiber, FR (1973) *Sybil: The true story of a woman possessed by sixteen separate personalities.* Chicago: Henry Regney Company.

Thorne, B (1998) *Person-Centred Therapy and Christian Spirituality: The secular and the holy.* Whurr: London.

West, C (1999) *First Person Plural: My life as a multiple.* New York: Hyperion Books.

Whitman, W (1855) A noiseless, patient spider. In H Rosengarten and A Goldrick-Jones (eds) (1993) *The Broadview Anthology of Poetry* (p. 301). Ontario: Broadview Press.

CHAPTER 9

DIAGNOSIS, STUCKNESS AND ENCOUNTER: EXISTENTIAL MEANING IN LONG-TERM DEPRESSION

RICHARD WORSLEY

In [the medical] model, the client is treated as a representative of a group of people who have been allocated a certain psychiatric diagnosis. It is from the psychiatrist's knowledge, according to research and other professional experience, of what is best for most people belonging to this diagnostic group, that the psychiatrist is an expert on what is best for an assumed representative of this group of people.

(Sommerbeck, 2005: 110)

INTRODUCTION

This is a case study of Emma, a university lecturer aged twenty-nine, with whom I worked for three and a half years, in the context of a university counselling service. In this setting long-term work is rare. She presented with a fairly intractable depression. She had received psychiatric care since the age of seventeen. Neither prolonged psychiatric treatment nor counselling has completely relieved her of her symptoms. My work with Emma is of profound interest to me on four grounds. The purpose of this chapter is to explore these four aspects of our work together and to reflect upon the links between them. Our work has been characterised by four themes:

1. Emma has been depressed for twelve years, and my three years' work with her has not ended the depression. I am aware of a circling through stuckness. I experience this on a small scale with many clients, but with Emma, as with a few other clients, this stuckness seems disproportionately difficult.

2. Emma has been in fairly constant psychiatric care for twelve years, mainly on an out-patient basis, but at the beginning as an in-patient with some symptoms of psychosis. The diagnosis of depression is a major label with which Emma lives. Her life-issues have been medicalised, and this she has found useful. Yet the stuckness is, from my perspective, associated in part with the label. This has produced in me strong feelings of hope for a version of Emma that might escape the strictures of diagnosis. (See Martin Buber's concept of confirmation of the client's potential, Kirschenbaum and Henderson, 1990: 41–63.) My own reactions to Emma are both complex and an important aspect of therapy. I have included in this chapter a brief, phenomenal description of my looking

back on our work during the early part of the process of writing.

3. Emma not only believes her diagnosis but also believes, at least tacitly, in the act of diagnosis. I do not. I decided, well into therapy, to confront this issue with Emma, in a way that I would not normally reveal my opinions to a client. I ceased, in other words, to be willing to work only within her frame of reference. This deserves some examination.

4. It is always pleasant to write about the client who, after a while, says that he feels better and need not come to counselling any more. That can be celebrated. Emma, after three years and more (and twelve of psychiatry!) is not 'cured'. However, the concept of cure is part of the mythology of the medical model. Perhaps we are never just 'cured' of our states of mind, distress or human experience. Emma may always be depressed. I think probably not, but there can be no guarantees. Therefore, far from being some sort of failure or disappointment on my part (and how that could harm the client!) Emma brings me face to face with the insights of positive psychology. Is it not possible for her, as a depressed person, to live both contentedly and creatively with whatever her life may bring in the future? Psychology and psychotherapy have so much more to offer than cure. At the heart of human growth is a deep existential well-being that transcends personal distress.

EMMA

Emma lectures in medieval and renaissance English and is single. She returned from her doctoral studies in the United States four years ago, to take up her current post. When she was seventeen years old, she experienced what she calls her 'nervous breakdown', being hospitalised for a number of weeks. Since her return to England, she has been under the care of a psychiatrist, diagnosed with clinical depression, with attendant panic attacks, and, in days gone by, quite a bit of obsessive-compulsive behaviour. She has been treated with antidepressants, beta-blockers and from time to time low doses of antipsychotics.

It has been a conscious decision of mine to remain with Emma through this long journey. Fewer than two per cent of my clients engage in long-term therapy with me in the university counselling service. My decision to work long-term with Emma was based on three perceptions on my part. We had a good working relationship. I liked her. This seemed to be reciprocated. However, she also brought out in me a stubborn streak, as if I was facing some sort of destructive force (or perhaps viewpoint, perspective) so that I felt myself to be allied with the creative configurations of Emma against the stuck and the diagnosed and ensnared. Finally, in supervision, I came to recognise that I believed in her ability to live creatively, and that much of her did not believe this. I felt that I could engage therapeutically with her creative side and was totally unwilling to desert her.

She gave her consent to my writing this case study. It is anonymised while remaining about the Emma that I came to know. In supervision, I came to recognise that writing

99

this would form a significant part of the end of her work with me. I will ask her to read through what I am writing, to change whatever she wants, and to understand that she may withdraw from this project at any time.

Emma and I share a rich and complex mixture of similarities and differences. One of these has proved to be a strange coincidence which as been an important part of therapy. Emma completed her doctoral studies at the University of Virginia with the distinguished medievalist, Professor Tony Spearing. Thirty-two years ago, I completed an English degree in which Tony Spearing was my Director of Studies. To understand and love the power of the imagery of medieval poetry has been a shared pursuit, and one that informs much of the imagery of Emma's terror.

DIAGNOSIS AND THE MEDICAL MODEL

Pete Sanders (2005) has argued cogently that diagnosis is anti-therapeutic because it ensnares the experience of the client as a whole person in the rhetoric of medicalisation: of broken brains cured by drugs alone. Of course, his stance does not preclude the concept that there are organic and genetic components to mental distress, for that might be to fly in the face of scientific evidence. (He does, however, doubt that such components exist; personal correspondence, 2006.) Rather, it is the medicalisation of distress which he opposes. This anti-reductionist stance has a long and important history from early luminaries such as Ivan Illich and RD Laing through to today's psychologists and psychiatrists who question the whole diagnostic materialism of conventional psychiatry (Bentall, 2003; Read, Mosher and Bentall, 2004; Jamison, 1994; Freeth, 2004). Paul Wilkins (2005) has set out briefly how distress can be conceptualised in a way that is compatible with person-centred thinking. Challenging Sanders' principled stance is the position of someone like Lisbeth Sommerbeck (2005) who has chosen to work within the context of orthodox psychiatry and looks for a complementarity between the two models: the medical model and the person-centred model. Yet, however Sanders and Sommerbeck may disagree in terms of tactics, they agree on the fundamental principle that human distress is to be accompanied and not pathologised.

Within the tradition of critical psychology, diagnosis is brought sharply into question. Bentall (2003) explores in depth the notion that diagnosis, as conventionally practised, is based upon an incoherent model of mental distress: it is seen as a physical disease. It is not. If I have influenza this can be categorised according to my symptoms, but also according to the precise properties of the virus which holds me in its grip. Bentall suggests that mental 'illnesses', by contrast, do not manifest as discreet entities; they only seem so because psychiatry constructs them to be thus. They are better seen as constellations of causal factors which can be clumped together only very approximately and which are unique to each individual.

In the light of this it would seem sensible to take conventional diagnosis with at least half a pinch of salt, and to listen carefully to the client as a person—of this I am sure. The problem is that life turns out to be not that simple. Many of our clients come to counselling with a mental health diagnosis. I recall the young girl who was attending a specialist eating disorders unit to help with the symptoms but who, after a course of initial group therapy, wanted to come to me to talk, as she put it, about the 'real' issues in her life. I recall the client who had experienced two severe bereavements and, after three months of speaking to no one about them, became acutely depressed. The psychologist had told her that he thought she might be bipolar, but she did not yet quite fit, so he, the professional, was puzzled!

The issue at stake with Emma was that she really valued her diagnosis, and my calling it into question was threatening. To be labelled as depressed absolved her of so much guilt! Her internal logic was that, since her experience was unacceptable to her family, she must either be wicked or ill. The latter was infinitely preferable. My working hypothesis—that Emma was distressed but not ill in the way we get sick with influenza, that the medical model version of depression is false—was apparently a direct contradiction of Emma's experience and world-view. How was I to respond to her and to myself?

I begin to answer this from the end rather than the beginning of therapy. The writing of this chapter has affected both Emma and me. I want to record my experience of reviewing her notes.

FIRST RETROSPECT

Today, as I read Emma's notes I felt the slightly bored apprehension of a writer with a job to get under way. I needed to organise my writing … I had other deadlines pressing on me. Then I read the notes which are just brief hints of around a hundred meetings with Emma. She said it was fine for me to write about her. I could simply observe that clients are often willing to take this risk because it might help others. Yet, deep down, I recognise the enjoyment I have in Emma's hopeful altruism. It is often there these days. The light by which I read shifted within me as I felt a growing wave of affection for the young woman who had allowed me to accompany her on this journey of more than three years. My first retrospect is that she is a precious human being and that my emotion and my stubbornness have stood out against her continuous self-deprecation.

I am astonished at the force and richness of my emotion. It feels as if I am looking for the first time at nearly the whole journey, which is just a few weeks from completion—at least with me. The travelling has felt rocky and so painful at times. I can feel particular compassion for her suffering because, after a long time together, she is for me an engaging and complex person. In her there is Otherness with which to dance. I admire her courage, even when it allows her to conceal in therapy the depth of her depression.

Beneath a sense of engaged affection lurks a sense of shock. I suddenly feel incompetent. The opening few sessions contained so much of what I had come to see as important about Emma. I knew so much so soon, but did not *understand* it! It had done no good just to have a cognitive grasp. Emma's speed of talking and of processing, whilst they defended her against being wrong, also shielded me from a full and emotionally

101

rooted insight of what it was like to be her. (And me—what had I contributed to this distance, this not-hearing?)

Gradually, I let myself become aware through the discomfort of this felt-incompetence that the therapy had twisted and turned as she and I wrestled over meaning. *Facts* had been there from near the beginning, but not meaning. The journey was interspersed with her fear—and then, time and again, a moving beyond it to new and emerging patterns. The meaning of it all emerged so slowly, because I guess it had to be a shared meaning in which she and I could hope. Diagnosis is not a shared meaning: it is imposed, even if it is an imposed comfort, an escape from the jolt of guilt. My felt-incompetence (how could I have known so much so early and to no effect?) is a mirror of the issue of diagnosis. While Emma had decided that it was better to be officially depressed than guilty I had to stay with an unknowing until the time emerged in Emma for a gradual, shared recognition. That is why diagnosis does not work. It knows too much—or not enough—too soon.

And as I read, I continued to feel hope for her future. I felt a cautious anticipation that she would read of my hope for her and that she would not try to render it irrelevant, discounted. I continue with a sense of the vulnerability of the whole process and the centrality of my capacity to use both affection and stubbornness towards, or even over against, Emma. Therapists' second-best resource is their very selves. The best is the client.

In these reactions to my overview of Emma's work with me, I am struck by the fact that it is the combination of positive feelings and hope towards Emma, together with the turmoil of wrestling with her own distorted, diagnosed self-image, which is the springboard for true encounter and for positive therapy with someone whose depression seems—and may be—intractable.

THE JOURNEY: THEMES AND PROCESS

Reading my notes of more than three years' work with Emma presents a problem. Most of what was said is lost. This sort of case study is very different from that of a single session recorded word for word (see Levitt, Chapter 14, this volume). What I am left with is my own summary of the therapy (albeit that this has been checked out with Emma at some length) both in the latter part of the therapeutic process itself and as part of the writing of this chapter. This summary is unashamedly interpretative in that I can no longer sort 'the facts' from my understanding of them. (On philosophical grounds I doubt that such a distinction can ever be fully made in any case.) My account of my journey with Emma, although recognisable to her, is *mine*. I offer it fairly briefly as a mixture of key themes and my understanding of the underlying process of the therapy. Often others will want to ask: What did you say to her? Draw the camera closer! It is precisely this that is lost. A thematic account is all that remains.

Herein is a dilemma for all therapists. I had a friend and colleague who records eighty per cent of all of his client work, and listens to all of it at least once. I have never done this, except as a training exercise. My friend will not lose the immediacy of and interventions. By contrast, I process 'how it is' in a very different form. I commitment, but would finally be overwhelmed attempting to emulate it. I aim to sharpen my awareness of work by an ongoing reflection upon a thematisation of both content and process. Sometimes I may deceive myself, but the pay-off is in having a compact grasp of what (I think) is happening in therapy. How therapists resolve this dilemma (precise recall versus internally processed, compact grasp) is a matter of personality. What follows is my own, idiosyncratic appreciation of how therapy works. Neither my friend nor I is right. Each person has to learn how to listen to their own work.

SELF-IMAGE

On bad days, Emma still feels that she is short and dumpy with uneven teeth. When I first met her I saw a young woman who was auburn-haired, pretty and with a slight lisp— yet her eyes stared out in fear. Many clients are afraid of beginning counselling but perhaps I did not appreciate anything of the depth of fear which Emma can experience. In spite of this disorientating fear, Emma could identify herself as being in quest of an identity. At school, she had been bullied (fat and short, she thought) and was bookish. By now academic success was her safest identity for she could rely on it over against the opinions of others.

At first I listened as intently as I could. Yet it felt like being overwhelmed with facts. On looking back I am still astonished at Emma's ability to project so much material about herself while being very scared and panicky. I wondered how she did it. It is perhaps that psychiatric care teaches clients to give a good account of themselves in a short space of time. Emma can own this idea in retrospect. However, I have come to see her ability to talk fluently and at great speed also as a defence. Being defensive is another important part of Emma's self-image: 'If I talk a lot, and at speed, I will not be accused of getting it wrong, because they will be shut out.'

I heard much of seemingly useful facts. What I missed was the implications of the process. The more I let Emma talk, the more I was complicit in being shut out: a 'them' like the rest of the world. It was a lot later in therapy that I was able to get in touch with how frustrated, impatient and overwhelmed I felt. I quietly and calmly asked her to listen to herself. 'Slow it down! Let yourself feel what you are saying!' This is not being directive (except in a very local way) but rather is about bringing my eclipsed self into the encounter. I needed her to stop and I claimed that for myself. The result was three-fold. Emma could articulate for the first time her knowledge of her defence and hence engage with it as meta-language (Rennie, 1998, Chapter 8). This gave her a new form of access to her behaviour and self-image. She did choose to slow down, and became more confident in hearing her feeling process. This turned out to be a piece of real acceptance on my part in that she experienced my desire for her to hear herself, not as directive, but as a willingness to accept what she felt. She then went on to experiment in life beyond therapy—with being heard by being less defensive.

GUILT AND FAMILY

Emma regarded her family as bizarre. She could say this from quite early on in therapy. However, I think, on reflection, that I was expected to hear this as an admission that she too was bizarre. (Emma is quite old-fashioned in her taste for entertainment—pubs, archery and dancing—and often recycled this part of her identity as evidence of her bizarreness. Because I have refused to collude in this she has come to see this aspect of herself as something that is her choice and of real value, part of being a unique person.) Her self-image, the role of her family and the role of guilt combined into a vicious Gestalt of self-condemnation—reinforced by Emma's ever-present internal critic.

Emma's maternal grandmother had been badly abused as a child, both physically and sexually. Her fear of living manifested itself through both depression and a series of outlandish behaviours that still haunt the succeeding generations. Grandma could make them feel bad like no-one else! Emma's mother had spent most of her life being depressed. By contrast, her father made little or no emotional contact with others. Emma came to wonder if he was to some extent autistic. Emma then became sandwiched between her mother's intermittent but deep depression, her father's inability to acknowledge Emma's feelings as real, and her younger sister's emotional demands upon the whole family.

At seventeen, Emma had become so depressed that she lapsed into deeply obsessive-compulsive routines while also losing a very real sense of herself in intermittent psychosis. However, it was not so much the fact of what she termed her 'madness' as the interminable guilt that became manifest in her relationship with me and others. For many months the subject of the family could be talked about only in a limited way. She felt guilty— *was* guilty. If she had become ill, then this must have harmed her mother. If she had become ill, then no wonder her father could not understand her. Her diagnosis seemed to her a relief—'People who are ill cannot be to blame'. But this did not work because the myth persisted. Emma had to feel guilty or the rest of her family would be brought into question.

I experienced this locked-in process as claustrophobic. I decided at about the halfway point in therapy to briefly take a more didactic role than usual. She and I had developed the metaphor of the 'beach ball of guilt'. Emma often pictured her family as sitting around the meal table. This stressed the unbearable nature of belonging there. I introduced Emma to a single idea: that what goes wrong is not only inside people but also between people (Laing and Esterson, 1964). We pictured guilt as a beach ball. Each member of the family passed it round like some furious and terrifying game of pass-the-parcel. Why did the ball end up with Emma? The benefit of this systemic view is that nobody is necessarily to blame for the dysfunction in a whole system.

This cognitive challenge was a precursor to the major challenge of the therapy, the function of Emma's diagnosis. I experienced time and again the entrapment of her self-image in her psychiatrist's description of her as an 'ill' person. She had no room to stand. She was rendered helpless. Depression is not an illness, but a want of meaning (Bentall, 2003). There came the point in the last half of therapy when I could no longer tolerate collusion with this as the sole interpretation of Emma's feelings. It felt like arm-wrestling her. She would not let me have my version of depression. It was an ongoing battle; I had to beware; it could be pursued too vigorously. It is enough for her to know that there are two versions of the story in the room. It would be wrong to deprive her forcibly of her diagnosis, which both frees and ensnares her! There was a lightness to the meeting over a frank disagreement handled with good humour. It is important to recognise in my standing over against Emma that I was not engaged in a cognitive disputation per se; I had little to gain from winning the argument. Rather, I wanted her to know that there was an alternative version of the story in the room.

SHAME

Emma's guilt sits on the surface. It is loud and obtrusive at times. There were groups of sessions of therapy in which the cognitive challenge I outline above would have been wholly inappropriate. In listening to Emma's description of herself, and in particular her compulsions and panic attacks, I became aware that what I was tending to miss was the profundity of her sense of shame. Shame is acutely different from guilt. It erodes the very core of being (Pattison, 2000):

> Shame itself is an entrance to the self. It is the affect of indignity, of defeat, of transgression, of inferiority and of alienation. No other affect is closer to the experienced self. None is more central to the sense of identity. Shame is felt as an inner torment, a sickness of the soul. (Kaufman, 1985: ix–x)

Emma was profoundly ashamed of who she was. I struggled in the face of her guilt and of the defensive pace of her words to find a presence to encounter her shame. I am struck only by the fact that there were moments when a loving look seemed to penetrate the shamefulness. The rebuilding of acceptance within her, and between us, was a long process. A stillness in being with Emma seems, in retrospect, to be its cornerstone.

Shame was intrinsic in Emma's process. The guilt could be extricated—the shame was hidden and shunned. Only as the shame retreated, could Emma begin to admit that her family were objectively problematical, and then to begin to find anger towards her father in particular.

VIVID IMAGERY AND THE EXISTENTIAL

Throughout our three years and more together, Emma would return from time to time to her fear of hellfire. (This was not a religious standpoint but a remnant of religious and other experiences.) This was of particular difficulty for her as a lecturer in medieval and renaissance literature. From *Piers Plowman* to *Paradise Lost*, the poetry of the period is saturated in the imagery of divine condemnation. I wanted to convey to Emma that this imagery was known to me for I too had some acquaintance with this literature. Yet I wanted also to convey that the theme of condemnation as a psychological–existential gestalt was, far from being bizarre or even shameful, very important (Tillich, 1952/1980: 51–3). At first, I held some notion that if we talked of what was feared this would decontaminate it. It did not. One cannot remove reality by exorcising a metaphor!

105

Paul Ricouer's (1978/1986) magisterial study of the metaphor puts forward the thesis that metaphor is not at all mere decoration. Rather, it is a persistent image the interpretation of which is inexhaustible. For any metaphor there is always more that can be said of its potential for meaning. Ricoeur terms this the *surplus of meaning*. However, he goes on to claim that it is from this very *surplus* that existential meaning emerges. So it would prove with Emma.

Near the end of therapy, I commented with a sort of wry smile that I was surprised that Emma had chosen to specialise in medieval and renaissance literature. There was far less hellfire in the modern era. To my astonishment, Emma coolly observed that she preferred the risk of hellfire to the sterility of Samuel Beckett. In other words, at some point in the deep past she had already made a choice for meaning over absence of meaning. It is better to be terrified than to not exist. Moreover, it had been done symbolically, in exactly the way that Carl Rogers notes that we exclude from symbolisation that which we cannot bear to experience fully (Rogers, 1951, Proposition IX: 503–7). She could begin to intuit a major part of her adult, professional life as a seeking after wholeness. This is the point of positive psychology. Even fear can be a highly functional choice: an existential commitment in which life begins.

THE ENDLESS CIRCLING OF DEPRESSION

My astonishment at how much I had learned cognitively about Emma in the first few sessions, and how useless that had proven to be, pointed to the fact that she was prone to circle repetitively through the same material time and again. This could test my patience. On reflection, this cyclical process is itself a manifestation of the actualising tendency. The process of therapy involves a retelling of the narratives that constitute our identity until, through a dialogue between the emotional structure and the underlying affect patterns, life's meanings shift. My challenge to Emma's story about the nature of her depression contributed to such a shift. The circling through material, so difficult to remain with at times, is the organism's provision for the possibility of this shift. It is when difficult material is repressed rather than circled through that stuckness occurs.

As a result of my challenging Emma's medical model version of depression a disjunct entered into the conversation: I think *but* I feel … I am increasingly intrigued by the question of what is in the matrix of the conversation, what is between two people rather than within either of them. There are objects of speech which exist in the interpersonal matrix as if independent of any one speaker. Between Emma and myself had grown the notion that thinking and feeling were not the same thing. Neither of us rationally believed that they were the same, of course. It was that this disjunct had become psychologically active. Emma was now able to engage with me in talking about her feelings as well as her, at times self-confessedly, dysfunctional thinking patterns. In interpersonal speaking new patterns emerge and voids cease. Thus, I recognised that the story of her madness had to be retold, perhaps time and again, until it took on a more functional shape. Yet, the diagnosis had it locked inside Emma in a particular way: 'Brains just go wrong; it's about serotonin; you do not need to feel guilty; it was not your fault, Emma'.

Stories are crucial to our identity. Emma seemed to have two stories. One condemned her to unspeakable guilt and shame. The other was that she was medically ill and hence could comfort herself over against the guilt. Diagnosis is a story. It is one that notoriously lacks meanings for the individual life, for as Lisbeth Sommerbeck pointed out in the quotation at the head of this chapter, diagnoses are not personal enough to contain *our* stories. I had to listen to Emma and me recycling her story before it could begin to work. The very act of recycling (seemingly so futile on the surface) is the royal route to new meaning. The ability for the client to envisage and engage with new meaning is a sign of journey's end. The accompanying therapist can be internalised.

SIGNS OF JOURNEY'S END

Emma and I know that there can be no guarantee that her depression will finally depart. However, Emma is now preparing to move on. In part, this is because she will be taking up a new post elsewhere in the next academic year. In part, it is because there are signs of new growth in Emma which may be sufficient for the day. Journey's end is signalled in a number of ways.

In the process of applying for her new job Emma had to face the question of whether she wanted to be seen as a disabled candidate. This is a very different label from the diagnosis and she was clear that she did not want this. It felt curious that the not-wanting was itself a mixed blessing from my perspective, even aside from the practical issues. Emma rejected the use of the label 'disabled' because it felt guilt-provoking. Was she taking advantage, hiding behind a diagnostic label? While this question is still very much part of her guilt pattern it also brings into question her trust of such labels. For whatever reason, she wanted to live as herself. Again, the question of labels is neither pure nor simple. Her motivation was still subject to guilt, yet the direction it was taking seemed to have greater sense of her being herself. When we are in transition there is no pure motivation. Functional and dysfunctional motivation can shade into each other. I felt and expressed my enjoyment at her challenging a label, whilst affirming the pragmatic utility of that label if she wanted to use it. She is experiencing a greater choice about labels.

The second sign of her moving on is that she has been able to talk with a new freedom about her family (see Rogers, 1957). There have been no restrictions as to her feelings about the complexity of living with them, or about her ambivalence towards their loving toxicity. Above all, she feels less integrated with her picture of her mother—who she wants to protect. Her emergent anger, although quite mild, places her mother at a sufficient distance for Emma recognise with certainty that she has her own individual identity and is not merely a place-holder within a family matrix.

DISCUSSION

A re-reading of Pete Sanders' (2005) passionate analysis of the need to oppose the medicalisation of distress, or of Bentall's (2003) deconstruction of mental illness, or of Laing and Esterson's (1964) analysis of madness as a construct and projection of family systemic dysfunction, can lead to a sense of outrage that so much human distress is abused by the medical model. It is a necessary part of our identity as person-centred therapists that we maintain in awareness those facts so well established in the United States and in Europe by the Soteria project (Read, Mosher and Bentall, 2004) and by the work of Garry Prouty and others (Prouty, Van Werde and Pörtner, 2002), namely that even extreme forms of psychotically-exhibited distress are resolvable through accompaniment, increased contact with self and encounter with an Other (Schmid, 1998). What is at stake is our authority, in a world in which cognitive-behavioural therapy is in the ascendant—and the pathologisation of distress is the order of the day. (I do not equate these two, except that they are both felt by person-centred practitioners as threats: challenges to our professional identity and credibility.) Therefore, I applaud in principle the insistent claim that mental health does not conform to the medical model and that diagnosis is deceptive and radically impersonal and depersonalising.

However, diagnosis is, in another sense, all too personal. It enters the therapy room with the client on many occasions. When I worked as a counsellor in medical general practice I was all too aware that the expectations set up by the doctor were inherited by therapeutic process, for good or ill. Emma's diagnosis of depression was an important object in her life. She was attached to it. It provided her with safety. To use her psychiatric diagnosis as she did is evidence of her actualising tendency. That which was handed to her on a plate she could recycle to protect herself from the depth of fear, guilt and shame which she experienced. Here is a dilemma. Sanders states the dilemma clearly: the tension between imposed and owned diagnosis:

> State-funded diagnoses, culturally-approved diagnoses, handed-down-in-the-family diagnoses, etc. but only one can really be fit for its purpose, that's the personally chosen, personally-managed diagnosis. I am 'against' state/cultural diagnoses on political grounds and will fight the structures which impose them, I am 'against' family (and other interpersonal) diagnoses on therapeutic/developmental grounds and will live with them as an inevitable consequence of being a social human. Personal diagnoses, I largely celebrate. (Sanders, personal communication, 2006)

However, Emma's diagnosis did not do its job particularly well, I suspect because it too was ensnared in the ambivalence and double-binds of her family. Her grandmother had bombarded the women of the next two generations with conflicting messages. Both had reacted with depression, while the menfolk simply escaped from feelings at all in various forms of ingrained emotional dysfunction. The sense of conflict and imposed responsibility was scarcely bearable since, at heart, Emma's was also a loving family. Yet, beneath these obvious conditions of worth lay the bedrock of a different sort of double bind. Because no-one else could be blamed for the situation, anger was not on the menu. Instead, the injunction to be silent with those who were either just as wounded as oneself or who were emotionally unrewarding generated an awful choice. Can one live with the toxic, or does one have to see oneself as toxic? The latter was very destructive for Emma, but it was an unconscious choice that would seem difficult to avoid.

Therefore one of the challenges of the therapy, from my point of view, was to find a tenable relationship with the diagnosis. At times, I had the sense that her psychiatrist was in the room with me. I became aware of the possibility of becoming the strident apostle for person-centred common-sense. The struggle I could have conceived as a struggle for Emma's soul. My metaphor I use deliberately. The medieval imagery of damnation ran through much of the work. The medieval world, as it is expressed in such works as *Piers Plowman,* is a world of black and white, or good and evil. This is about splitting and projection. It would have been tempting to have marked off the diagnosis and the psychiatrist as bad, when in fact it was quite functional for Emma in some ways, albeit limited ones.

Throughout, I used the image within me of keeping in the room an alternative version of Emma's story about herself. Although she may feel that I was over-challenging at times, my aim was always to offer the alternative without wanting to encroach upon her legitimate defences. Her view of her world is important; sacrosanct. It was never my job to overcome it, to convince her otherwise, but rather to create an environment, a set of possibilities through which she could explore her own ability to be a depressed swan, beautiful and creative. We started off with different stories of what afflicted Emma and moved towards each other. In our last two sessions, I sat with a self-confessed sense of smugness and enjoyed her version of her family and her anger that I could recognise as wholly real and appropriate.

In therapy, clients tell and retell their stories until a version emerges which is more functional than the starting point. My chief learning, from reviewing my work with Emma for this case study, has been my coming to understand that stories are recycled over long periods of time in a particular and fascinating way. My not understanding and Emma's not understanding seem to have danced hand in hand. Time and again, the pattern of groups of sessions could be seen as two people negotiating meaning that neither had possessed until then. Emma would make available to both of us versions of her story which resonated with what had gone before. The too and fro of sessions began to represent our shared search for meaning.

How, then, have I come to see Emma's diagnosis and my relation with it? I am sure that it would have been wrong—incongruent—for me to collude with the diagnosis by failing to challenge Emma's view of herself as merely ill. Not least because (although this was her consciously held belief and category) she did not live by it. The guilt remained strong. Therefore I needed also to empathise with that other configuration which, wanting to take on too much responsibility, sought out meaning. At times, I could feel the temptation within myself to be too strident about my own world view. I needed to find a balance within myself between being present to Emma and, simultaneously, keeping another version of the story in the room. I maintained a tension of meanings, which is

109

one way of describing the meeting of two people at depth. For Emma the diagnosis was the product of her attempt to actualise a version which was, in many ways, functional for her. She had found it a mighty relief to be less to blame! It was also a restriction upon her further growth because it kept trapped within its own category the potential for her to generate meaning about her life, her depression, her family and, above all, herself as a deeply worthwhile and lovely human being. In a sense, it turned out to be my task to create enough ambivalence about the diagnosis for Emma to meet, in me, a number of versions and thence evolve for herself a version of her own story more functional than the old one. Thus, therapy is dialogue. The outcome is spontaneous, unconsciously evolving from the 'negotiations' of client and therapist.

When individual experience is labelled, categorised, generalised by the medicalisation of distress, then the therapeutic dialogue needs to engage this object-in-the-room. This social construction of distress is a way that allows, through empathy and challenge, the client to create meaning. The therapist cannot impose meaning, but the therapist who is too shy about their own frame of reference may well inhibit the dialogical capacity of the client's creativity.

But what meaning? Emma's metaphor of herself as a depressed swan is powerful and yet provisional. Neither of us knows who it is that she is becoming. It is the act of becoming which is functional. The characteristic insight of positive psychology (Joseph and Worsley, 2005) is that the human growth which flows from client-/person-centred/positive therapy is a true enhancement of human living, far more than the mere relief of symptoms. Kay Redfield Jamison (1994) gives a challenging and beautiful account of the author's engagement with her own bipolarity, through which she comes to value her experience in spite of her suffering, while exploring the relevance of bipolar disorder to artistic and poetic creativity, and while holding down her demanding job as a professor of psychiatry at Johns Hopkins University School of Medicine. Her view of her distress is rather more conditioned by the medical model than I would like. Nevertheless, she has a clear view of its positive nature. It cannot be said to contribute to her happiness in a superficial sense. Positive psychology is not superficial. Happiness is about a depth of well-being in the face of, and even because of, diagnosis and painful adversity.

In Emma, is the positive real? I can certainly point to an alleviation of some symptoms. Over time, Emma has moved away from madness and from the fear of madness, although the latter is by no means complete yet. She has moved away markedly from her obsessional-compulsive behaviours and, to a lesser extent, from her panics. She has learned that panic, however unpleasant, is rather more functional and a lot less shameful than she once thought. Her suicidal ideation is diminished both in frequency and in intensity. Her guilt is still a problem but may well be diminishing further. But all of that is essentially the language of diagnosis, however welcome the relief might be. What more is there?

The reply needs to be Emma's. I have only my version. I am fascinated by the richness of the image of the depressed swan. Swans are indeed lovely creatures. Where I live I can walk and see them at will. They manifest a serenity on the surface which combines elegantly with power, and even struggle, beneath the surface. They are social, faithful, and good parents. They are independent and intelligent creatures.

True growth begins to evolve a uniqueness which expresses some depth of the individual's personhood. I can begin to glimpse what this is in Emma. She has a forthright pride in her personal values. She struggles with not conforming to some perceived social norms but does not try to conform, and is willing to become angry with any criticism of her for this. She is creating a distance between her mother and herself, in terms of not experiencing the need to protect her mother by distorting her own anger at the conditionality which her family puts onto her. Her description of her family feels increasingly guilt-free—and real. She is increasingly able to hope in the face of her depression that, even if there is no major remission of symptoms, her life can have shape and purpose. Above all, she has developed the insight that even fear is a worthwhile, temporary cost to pay for having meaning in life. It is better to 'believe' in Dante than Beckett. Thus the seed of future-orientation is affirmed in present awareness.

But of 'swan-ness', Emma herself would have to say what she is coming to see in her own being.

CONCLUSION

I want to offer final comments about the four elements of this case which I identified at the beginning of the chapter as important.

1. *Emma's stuckness.* It would be too easy to blame the diagnosis or even Emma's psychiatrist for her stuckness. She had, after all, been rendered dependent upon her conception of herself as depressed. However, this is far too simplistic. Emma is stuck, or at least is moving far more slowly towards an acceptable-to-her level of functionality than many clients. This stuckness is for me best conceptualised in terms of the internal dynamics, of which Emma's diagnosis is but one. I note Mearns and Thorne's (2000) comment that configurations have the tendency to accrue to themselves that which confirms their view of life and, consequently, to reject that which challenges that view. Rogers, of course, had said the same thing about the whole person (Propositions X – XII, Rogers, 1951: 498–509). The theory of configurations of self adds to this that it is each configuration which has this defensive capacity:

> An additional means for the accrual of other elements relates to the *self-fulfilling* nature of configurations. Once a configuration actively participates in the existential life of the person it can bring about its own narrative, hence adding elements to expand its existence and veracity. (Mearns and Thorne, 2000: 118. Original emphasis)

It seems to me that a number of configurations had emerged in Emma which conspired to keep her stuck. These might include a Good Daughter, who must take the blame for the suffering in the family; a Woman in the family, who must be responsible for all feelings while being thoroughly disapproved of by the men in the family; the Geek, who is odd rather than creative; a Sick Person, who is at least absolved of guilt so long as she does not challenge the notion of guilt; the Guilty Person, who must keep feeling the guilt in order to absolve others. With those who are chronically depressed the pattern is deeply embedded in the structure of self that has evolved. Therapy is a bit like unpicking a tangled ball of wool. It requires determination and patience but, above all, the therapist must not be sucked into the illusion of hopelessness.

2. *The perniciousness of the medical model* is that it deprives experience of the possibility of meaning. For Emma this has a short-term pay-off within the economy of configurations outlined above. However, there is a broader issue here than the mere shortcomings of the medical model. While Richard Bentall (2003) has produced a magisterial deconstruction of the medical model from the perspective of clinical psychology, the fault in the medical model is even more deep-rooted. The model blatantly ignores some of the key issues in the philosophy of the mind (Searle, 1998; Gray, 2004). In the medical model the mind is seen as a chemical-biological machine in which depression is *in fact and solely* about serotonin. This is to deny that the mind's brain generates meaning, and moreover that meaning affects the brain. If it does not, then either there is no meaning and no consciousness, or else the brain and mind are not truly associated but separate, as Descartes had believed. To work with Emma is to be faced over a long period with the need to have faith in meaning.

3. *Whose frame of reference?* To some person-centred therapists, my decision to state my own views in opposition to Emma's frame of reference is controversial. At least one reader of this chapter has said as much to me. It would be possible to burble on about congruence. But why did I decide to be congruent about this at the time I did? The challenge is a good enough one. For me the answer is two-fold. In order to offer not only understanding but also faith to that part of Emma which *is* for growth, I finally felt that I had to stand up against the configurations which conspired against growth. After some consideration, I came to the conclusion that on this occasion this required a cognitive challenge to the client (or some aspects of her). This is in part about empathy for the oppressed parts. However, it is also about encounter (Schmid, 1998). There has been far too little thought in the person-centred movement about what constitutes encounter. This would be a long discussion, out of place in this chapter. All I can do is to ask the reader to contemplate Rogers' words to Martin Buber:

> [I]f this client comes to the point where he can experience what he is expressing, but also can experience my understanding of it and *reaction to* it, and so on, then therapy is just about over. (Kirschenbaum and Henderson, 1990: 50)

Finally to conceal my reactions and beliefs would, in this case, have been wilfully anti-therapeutic. Part of any healthy person consists of their capacity to meet fully another person. Challenge is also part of encounter (Worsley, 2006).

4. *A positive psychology.* Emma has undergone quite a bit of change already. She is no longer obsessive-compulsive, except perhaps vestigially. She has fewer and less severe

panic attacks and she no longer regards these as shameful. She is beginning to have a realistic perspective upon the life of her family. Above all, she is able to see visits home as both enjoyable and also potentially a little toxic, and so requiring care. Nevertheless, let us suppose that she does not cease to experience symptoms of depression. For the medical model this would be a failure. (Whose?) Positive psychology offers another perspective completely (see Jamison, 1994). Positive psychology involves in its therapeutic practice the 'application of positive psychology research to the facilitation of optimal functioning' (Linley and Joseph, 2004: 4). If Emma were to remain depressed for the rest of her life, this would not prevent her from contacting her optimal functioning—for optimal is optimal for Emma not for any outside clinician. To cut a long story short, I suggest that the counsellor who can see the optimal (within the long-term distress or residual, intractable distress) is able to offer a hope, a love of life, which goes way beyond the burden of symptoms. The counsellor who, facing the apparently intractable, secretly despairs, is likely to take the client down with them. This I believe Emma and I have learned together and I am grateful to her for this.

The task seems to have been to create enough tension between Emma's view and mine to allow her to negotiate her own meanings, while being clear that I too hold meanings and values concerning mental distress. In this very process of meaning-generation, it becomes clear that client-/person-centred/positive therapy has the capacity to facilitate the client in growth which transcends the mere relief of symptoms, and involves a facing of those existential-spiritual questions which themselves begin to define the purpose, the directionality, of life.

POSTSCRIPT

Some ten months after I wrote the first draft of this case study, I came across a card that Emma had given me at the end of therapy. At first I looked at it with a general, warm affection. I opened it and again read the words. It was as if I had never read them before. In fact, I think I did not read them before. For Emma thanked me, amongst other things, for helping her see her distress in a new and creative way. I stand amazed that I had edited this out of my awareness—as though it were too much to hope for.

REFERENCES

Bentall, RP (2003) *Madness Explained: Psychosis and human nature.* London: Penguin.

Freeth, R (2004) A psychiatrist's experience of person-centred supervision. In K Tudor and M Worrall (eds) *Freedom to Practise: Person-centred approaches to supervision* (pp. 247–66). Ross-on-Wye: PCCS Books.

Gray, J (2004) *Consciousness: Creeping up on the hard problem.* Oxford: Oxford University Press.

Jamison, KR (1994) *Touched with Fire: Manic-depressive illness and the artistic temperament.* New York: Free Press.

Joseph, S and Worsley, R (2005) A positive psychology of mental health: A person-centred perspective. In S Joseph and R Worsley (eds) *Person-Centred Psychopathology: A positive psychology of mental health* (pp. 348–57). Ross-on-Wye: PCCS Books.

Kaufman, G (1985*) Shame: The power of caring*. Rochester, NY: Shenkman Books.

Kirschenbaum, H and Henderson, VL (eds) (1990) *Carl Rogers: Dialogues*. London: Constable.

Laing, RD and Esterson, A (1964) *Sanity, Madness and the Family*. London: Tavistock.

Linley, PA and Joseph, S (2004) *Positive Psychology in Practice*. Hoboken, NJ: John Wiley.

Mearns, D and Thorne, B (2000) *Person-Centred Therapy Today: New frontiers in theory and practice*. London: Sage.

Pattison, S (2000) *Shame: Theory, therapy, theology*. Cambridge: Cambridge University Press.

Prouty, G, Van Werde, D and Pörtner, M (2002) *Pre-Therapy: Reaching contact-impaired clients*. Ross-on-Wye: PCCS Books.

Read, J, Mosher, LR and Bentall, RP (2004) *Models of Madness: Psychological, social and biological approaches to schizophrenia*. Hove and New York: Brunner Routledge.

Rennie, DL (1998) *Person-Centred Counselling: An experiential approach*. London: Sage.

Ricoeur, P (1978/1986) *The Rule of Metaphor: Multi-disciplinary studies of the creation of meaning in language* (trans. R Czerny). London: Routledge.

Rogers,CR (1951) *Client-Centered Therapy*. London: Constable.

Rogers, CR (1957) A process conception of psychotherapy. In CR Rogers (1961/1967) *On Becoming a Person: A therapist's view of psychotherapy* (pp. 125–59). London: Constable.

Sanders, P (2005) Principled and strategic opposition to the medicalisation of distress and all of its apparatus. In S Joseph and R Worsley (eds) *Person-Centred Psychopathology: A positive psychology of mental health* (pp. 21–42). Ross-on-Wye: PCCS Books.

Schmid, PF (1998) Face-to-face—the art of encounter. In B Thorne and E Lambers (eds) *Person-Centred Therapy: A European perspective* (pp. 74–90). London: Sage.

Searle, J (1998) *The Mystery of Consciousness*. London: Granta Books.

Sommerbeck, L (2005) The complementarity between client-centred therapy and psychiatry: The theory and its practice. In S Joseph and R Worsley (eds) *Person-Centred Psychopathology: A positive psychology of mental health* (pp. 110–27). Ross-on-Wye: PCCS Books.

Tillich, P (1952/1980) *The Courage to Be*. New Haven, NY: Yale University Press.

Wilkins, P (2005) Assessment and 'diagnosis' in person-centred therapy. In S Joseph and R Worsley (eds) *Person-Centred Psychopathology: A positive psychology of mental health* (pp. 128–45). Ross-on-Wye: PCCS Books.

Worsley, RJ (2006) Emmanuel Levinas: Resource and challenge for therapy. *Person-Centered and Experiential Psychotherapies, 5*, 208–20.

CHAPTER 10

THE DERAILMENT OF A SPIRITUAL QUEST: THE CASE OF HANS SIEVEZ[1]

MARTIN VAN KALMTHOUT

INTRODUCTION

In this chapter I present a person-centered interpretation of the case of Hans Sievez, the protagonist of a best-selling Dutch novel *Kneeling on a Bed of Violets* (Siebelink, 2005). I will also describe some ideas about the therapy which I, as a person-centered therapist, would like hypothetically to offer him.

When I read the book for the first time it touched me intensely. That many other readers must have been similarly touched is demonstrated by the fact that, by the beginning of 2007, thirty-one editions had been published. But why was this so? No doubt the reasons are different for different readers. To me, the most shocking element in the book was the phenomenon of a child, born in bizarre circumstances, succeeding in freeing himself from these, but eventually repeating in later life the very things which he had set his face against so intensely. Maybe the most dramatic aspect of the story is that, in repeating the old pattern, he dragged with him not only his older son but also his wife, who at first had figured as a model of health compared to her morbidly addicted husband. In his second son the repetition is even more dramatic. This son he mistreats emotionally in the same way as his father once mistreated him—with all the terrible consequences implied.

I increasingly realized that what the author (Jan Siebelink) is describing is utterly timely. This is true not so much because there are still so many Christian sectarians (at least not in the Netherlands), but rather because all this is about a universal phenomenon. In our present world the phenomenon is most clearly present in so-called Muslim fundamentalism, but it is ageless and universal and can be found in all religions, ideologies and systems of belief. To summarize briefly: the phenomenon implies that somebody who is in a critical phase of his life (almost always the result of his personal past) comes under the influence of 'fanatic believers' in the broad sense of that word. These fanatics manipulate and indoctrinate him and seduce him into accepting extremes of thought and action. The protagonist of Jan Siebelink's novel fits this pattern completely.

---

1. This chapter is a translation of an article first published in *Tijdschrift Cliëntgerichte Psychotherapie* (van Kalmthout, 2007). I thank the editor of the journal for her permission to reprint the article in translation.

There is no doubt that psychologists will have their thoughts about the phenomenon described, but what about psychotherapists? Can they say something sensible about it? What would that be? The limits of such an enterprise are all too clear. In the past some psychotherapists analyzed a so-called 'case on paper'. A well-known example is the reflection on Ellen West by Carl Rogers (Rogers, 1980: 164–180). We know roughly as much about Ellen West as we do about the protagonist of Jan Siebelink's novel, Hans Sievez. This makes it possible to analyze the case and to imagine the way therapy might proceed. In fact the story of Hans Sievez is autobiographical in that the author describes in his book the true story of his father and the family of which the author is the older son. There is, however, a great difference between the two cases. Ellen West experienced several therapies in her life (which were criticized by Rogers), while Hans Sievez never participated in any therapy and, in all probability, would never have agreed to undergo therapy. In interviews, the author of the novel rejected with outrage every attempt to treat Hans Sievez as a psychiatric case.

Like the case of Ellen West, the case of Hans Sievez is well suited to illustrate one's approach to therapy: in the article by Rogers, for instance, his views on therapy become quite clear. Nevertheless, we don't know whether his analysis is right or whether his therapy would have been successful. The same is true for the possible therapy of Hans Sievez. In the following, I will risk illustrating how a person-centered approach to the case of Hans Sievez would appear, more or less. I accept that there are limits involved in such an endeavor.

LIFE HISTORY

In this section I give a fairly detailed description of the life history of Hans Sievez. Although I follow as accurately as possible the facts presented in the novel, it is not just a repetition of the story, but a selection and interpretation from my reading of it. In fact, I already start, in this section, the process of diagnosis, or what I consider as the core problem of this case.

Hans Sievez is the only son of a father who is a workman in a brickyard, in which he is allowed, to his annoyance, to work only in summer and in which he never gets a permanent job. Two elder brothers of Hans have worked in the same factory, but died through an accident at work. To his parents Hans is an afterthought and a very clingy child; a mother's boy. He is an asthmatic. His father mistreats him emotionally and physically and his mother is unable to prevent this. To make matters worse, his mother dies at young age leaving Hans alone with his father. He finds comfort with a girl friend (who he will marry as an adult) as well as with his little rabbit. He often escapes from his chill circumstances by going to a hiding place, built by himself, in the peat moor. It is remarkable that Hans compensates for his lack of love by putting on plays in the schoolyard to attract attention from his schoolfellows. When he discovers that his father has sold his beloved rabbit he decides to leave, never to return home.

What is of utmost relevance is that his father has come under the influence of boatmen who, convinced that the regular Christian Church preaches a totally false doctrine, have founded an extreme Christian sect. His father then becomes a member of that sect and, from then on, Hans and his mother have to go with him, against their will, to its services. Later on, these services are even held in the family's living room. At the funeral of Hans' mother one of the sect's preachers gives the sermon. Hans' father reads the Holy Bible to the family daily and he does so with an almost screaming voice. One day Hans finds his father outside with bloody lips. He does not recognize his son. He has had, so he says, some kind of encounter with God 'who had beaten him, had seized him by the scruff of the neck and had thrown him onto the earth'. Sometimes, Hans sees his father in the garden, mad and shouting that everything is rotten and that evil is in everything, even the plants. Hans grows fearful of his father and wants to leave home as soon as possible.

When the time comes, Hans leaves for the other side of the country to learn the trade of market gardener, in which he turns out to be very successful. What stands out in this period of his life is his struggle with his landlady, who tends to force all kinds of things on him. Although Hans is aware of this, he has the greatest difficulty in holding her at a distance. The same happens between Hans and a colleague, who tries to seduce him into becoming a member of a sect of the same kind as his father's. Here, the danger is that history will simply repeat itself. Hans turns out to be a person who is very gullible and easily seduced. In the beginning he is aware of what is happening and keeps the seducer at a distance. But later he yields. Hans is half-hearted in his rejection. There is a part of him that is not firm. Another part of this pattern is that, when he does resist, he can only do so by falling into the other extreme—a physical fight.

Many years later, when Hans is already married to the girlfriend of his youth and running his own nursery garden, his old colleague re-emerges and, whether he likes it or not, Hans increasingly comes under his influence. This process is due, in part, to the fact that, commercially speaking, the nursery garden is not very successful and also to the fact that Hans feels hurt and humiliated by some of his colleagues and wholesale dealers. It turns out that he grows increasingly sensitive to, and in need of, the message of his old friend, a message which apparently satisfies a deeply rooted need: 'the desire for what is hidden, that which is certain all the time'.

Meanwhile his wife notices that something strange is happening in Hans; something she has not previously noticed. She starts to be concerned about him and for the first time in their relationship an unresolvable conflict arises. What is important here is that Hans does not dare tell her anything about his religious interests but practises them in secret. He is afraid of a confrontation with her. She for her part tries everything to confront Hans about these matters. His own doubts result in him making several attempts to sever all connections with his new friends of faith. But eventually he comes more and more under their influence and loses contact with his wife. A religious experience that Hans undergoes in his nursery garden sets its seal on this. This experience has much in common with the one his father had in the parental home. From the moment of this religious experience, Hans feels himself to be one of the elect; a feeling which later on will be confirmed in an official meeting of the sect. In this community, Hans experiences

117

an enormous amount of approval and admiration because of what has occurred to him. He feels quite happy as a consequence, but he becomes even more alienated from all earthly things, especially from his wife and business. His older son, the writer of the present novel, Jan Siebelink, identifies strongly with his father and would be most happy to follow the same path. Father Hans condones this, but makes him swear to say nothing about it to his mother.

The second son of the family, unlike his brother, resists his father's religious faith. Furthermore, he indirectly questions his father's priorities as he does not feel loved by him. Notwithstanding his undeniable talents and his intimate relationship with his mother, his life comes to a troubled end. He fails at school and is even expelled several times because of misbehavior. He becomes an alcoholic and ridicules his father's faith in public.

Hans' wife fights a war to the death to make her husband change his mind. Her challenges are like water off a duck's back. She grows desperate. She and her children are forced by Hans to participate in a service at home of no less then two hours each Sunday morning. Then he reads the old texts and gives a sermon himself like his father had once done. Later on, they have to accept that the service is led by one of the leading preachers of the sect and that he and the other members not only drink coffee afterwards but also have dinner together. His wife gives in, though knowing better. Hans isolates himself more and more from his wife and children. He grows lonely and completely inaccessible. He lives in a different world and can no longer be held responsible for his actions and for what he neglects. His wife's state of health deteriorates. She makes herself give in to a course of events which is opposed to everything that is of value to her—and still the loss of her husband seems inevitable.

In a dream, Hans' father manifests himself and informs Hans that he is on the right track. In this way, so it seems, his father is still in control of him. The preachers, on their side, emphasize with the utmost seriousness that Hans better not think that salvation is already his. Hans, for his part, accepts that his wife and children will never be saved. Hans himself, convinced of his worthlessness and sinfulness, will be haunted until his death by his fear that eventually he too will be rejected.

During one of the Sunday services Hans' wife collapses. She is now sure that she does not want to accept the present situation any longer. She refuses Hans sexually and tells him that she is going to leave. One evening, when Hans arrives home very late because of his attending a service somewhere in the country, he discovers that she has left, taking with her the younger boy. She stays away for two weeks and is not willing to come back unless Hans breaks with the preachers once and for all. Although Hans asks himself whether God will forgive or reject him for this decision, eventually he decides to submit to her conditions. For five years he lives without any contact with the sect, but then the preachers start to visit him again in his nursery garden, and again Hans is unable to resist them. He is aware of his weakness and hates himself. He feels trapped by them and unable to escape their influence.

Another remarkable event takes place in this period. Hans falls in love with the wife of his older son. He fantasizes sexually about her and buys the kind of presents for her which only lovers give each other. His daughter-in-law is allowed to be closer to him than his own wife and sometimes it looks as if his wish to have a daughter instead of a second son is going to come true. In the meantime, the relationship with his second son deteriorates badly. One day he tells Hans in a very direct way that he is only concerned about his own salvation and is not interested in the fact that his wife and children are the victims of this addiction. To his own embarrassment, Hans says to him that it would have been better if he had not been born. For his son this is the definitive proof that his father has never accepted him.

On the day that the atheist parents of his new daughter-in-law come to meet him, Hans gives a speech which is much like a sermon. Although everybody is surprised, they admire Hans at the same time. Hans spews out, without any hesitation, one long sentence after the other and, quite remarkably, in the most beautiful, solemn and antique language. It looks as if Hans is transcending himself, talking in a kind of trance; inspired and without any sign of anxiety. He expresses in the most forceful way his deepest conviction. Although amongst those present only his older son shares his faith, everybody is deeply touched and impressed by Hans' performance.

Later on, Hans becomes ill. He turns out to be suffering from lung cancer. His condition deteriorates rapidly and the nursery garden has to be closed. When Hans is alone for a while with his daughter-in-law he asks her to ring one of the preachers to inform them about his condition, without saying anything to her mother-in-law. The preachers arrive immediately to take over. Nobody else, not even his wife and children, is allowed to come near him. Once again, Hans' wife is unable to throw them out and only after he has died (when the preachers have left) does she regain control.

It is remarkable that even on his sickbed Hans shows no interest whatsoever in his family. He seems to be concerned exclusively with his own salvation and is assisted in this by six anonymous preachers and two old friends from the sect. They continue to feed Hans' anxiety about his ultimate condemnation. They seem to believe themselves to have complete insight into God's ways. The absence of any kind of human or personal approach to the dying man is painful. Every sign of suffering on the part of the family is rejected in a chilly and coercive manner and on the basis of theological arguments. The most painful aspect of this is that Hans himself wants things to happen in this way, in spite of his physical and psychological exhaustion. While Hans is dying, his younger son is not present and nobody is able to find him. Later on, it turns out that he has been roaming about from one pub to the other.

At the end of the story, the older son says to his mother that he guesses it has been rather tough for her to live with his father. She flatly denies this saying that it was always alright between her and Papa. She expresses her hope that the younger son will return home soon and that she will meet Hans again in the hereafter.

DIAGNOSIS

In person-centered philosophy diagnosis is conceptualized differently than in psychiatry. Diagnosis is not about categorizing mental disorders in order to treat them in the right way, but about finding an answer to the question of the essence of the problems the client is struggling with.

Hans Sievez is struggling with a classical conflict: namely how to engage in a personal relationship without losing himself (van Kalmthout, 1997, 2002). In his adult life we see this conflict for the first time with his landlady. Hans is aware that she does not respect his boundaries and tries to keep her at a distance. He never succeeds completely and in the end only a definitive break brings about the solution. The same struggle is present between him and his sectarian friend and (following in his footsteps) between him and the other preachers. Hans' doubts are very intense in different consecutive phases, but in the end he has got the worst of it—he loses himself. Only in those periods during which he breaks completely with the other person does he succeed. The same conflict is present between Hans and his wife. Although he initially succeeds in attaching himself to her in a healthy way, he is not able to engage fully in conflict with her. Only by closing himself off emotionally from her is he able to follow his own path. In the conflict with his younger son he sees only one solution: to reject him in the same way he himself was once rejected by his father. With his older son, on the other hand, a kind of symbiotic relationship is formed in which the latter identifies with his father and wants to be like him. With such a relationship Hans has no problems. But in such a relationship there is no personal and direct contact either. It is the kind of relationship which happens between a leader and a follower.

Sometimes Hans is overcome by uncontrollable aggression. For instance, he strikes down his friend in the beginning of their relationship and later he does the same to one of his wholesale dealers who has hurt and humiliated him. Common to all these conflicts is that Hans either escapes from them or settles them by violence. He is not able to speak out clearly and honestly and thus settle the conflict in a satisfactory way. There is only fight or flight. Today we would say that something is wrong with his anger management. By his avoidance behavior he nurses, in silence, his hatred about the disappointments and humiliations until the cup is full and brimming over. When an outburst of rage follows it is completely out of proportion. The violence he uses in such a moment is a repetition of his father's mistreatment of him. Within gentle Hans a time bomb is ticking, put there by his father.

The background of this core conflict, which divides Hans inwardly, has to be found in his early youth. Physically speaking, he was not strong and his asthma was an expression of this. He is a mummy's boy who hides with her against the violence of his father. But, in fact, he is not secure with her; first of all because she is not able to protect him against his father and then because she dies at young age. In such a way Hans has had bad experiences of engaging in intimate relationships. Where his father is concerned, Hans almost perished physically and emotionally as a consequence of the relationship. In the relationship with his mother he experienced how risky it was to become attached to a beloved person since he lost her with the crushing finality of death. Hans had not learned in his youth to feel and to express what was going on within him, let alone to communicate openly and directly with others. Naturally he retreats into himself, keeps silent and fights conflicts in indirect ways. Thus, he grows more and more isolated and loses contact with reality.

In this critical situation little Hans was in search of a way out through several survival strategies. He started an intimate relationship with an animal, he built a hiding place in the peat moor and tried to attract attention by portraying himself as an actor. He also dreamt of having a future with his beloved wife and his own business through which he would be independent of everybody. When these dreams did not come to pass, he took flight into a new dream: religious salvation and election. Life is both too heavy and not enough for him. He is looking for something loftier.

The latter, in many respects, has the character of an addiction. In his discontent, he took flight into something that generated a temporary relief; something through which earthly misery can be transcended. And if this would not happen in this life, then, so he hoped, it certainly would happen in the future life, after death. It is characteristic of addiction that everything previously dear to him became of secondary importance and was even sacrificed. This is the case with many types of addiction. It is also characteristic of addiction that the many signs indicating the suffering of those things previously very dear to him—wife, children, business—are no longer noticed. At least, they are not permitted to touch him from within or determine the course of his action. Hans turned away from these warning signs in the same way as he turned away from the loving efforts of his wife to address him as a responsible and beloved person. Similarly, he did not allow himself to be touched by the childlike efforts of his younger son to gain his father's love.

From the perspective of person-centered philosophy Hans opted for the kind of meaning in life that is unhealthy, alienating and inauthentic (van Kalmthout, 2005, 2006). He failed to develop himself in an authentic way, starting from respect for himself. As he was not empathic and respectful towards himself he stayed caught in his old neurotic patterns or survival strategies which were now counterproductive. Logically, his relationships were colored by this. He treated himself and then others in the way that he was once treated. In his search into the meaning of life Hans Sievez had grown alienated from the reality of life. He looked for the meaning of life outside himself and his relationships. As he was not able to find it there, he took flight into a fundamentalistic form of religion in which there is no place for love or truth and in which everything is built around dogma and ritual-like anchor points for anxious people in search of moorings. Unfortunately, Hans was not able to find a healthy spiritual path—which could have helped him to overcome his existential crisis—without neglecting the core of all true religion and spirituality.

THERAPY

Hans Sievez lived in an era (approximately the first half of the twentieth century) in which it was highly improbable that he would have undertaken therapy. Nevertheless it is conspicuous that neither he, nor his wife or children, tried to find any kind of fitting help for the enormous problems with which the family struggled; for instance friends, a minister, the family doctor or one of the teachers. It is a measure of the degree to which the family had withdrawn into itself. There was a complete absence of any tendency to ask for help from anybody. Even if they had lived in current times, in which therapeutic help is much more accessible and taken for granted, their attitude would have prevented them from either seeking help or in making full use of any help offered to them. So the first problem was one of motivation.

Person-centered therapy starts with the premise that problems arise within relationships and that, because of this, they have to be solved within relationships. That is why the therapeutic relationship is crucial in this form of therapy. Within this basic assumption there is an enormous amount of freedom for the therapist. In person-centered terminology we could say that the cause of the problem of Hans Sievez is the fact that he experienced, in the course of his life, no empathy, respect or congruence. Therefore, the essence of the therapy should be that a place is created in which he is allowed to experience these three so-called 'core conditions' and to correct in such a manner the emotional damage that has occurred to him (van Kalmthout, 1997, 2002).

I examine the question of what I, as a therapist, would do in the event of Jan Sievez entering my therapy room. The first thing of importance to me would be to gain his confidence. A necessary condition for that would be to take him very seriously in all respects, including his bizarre behavior. This does not imply that I must agree with him in everything, but what it does imply is that I will make a committed and very honest effort to understand him without judgment. To formulate it in person-centered concepts: I would engage him empathically and respectfully. If it works out well this would give to Hans the feeling of not being rejected and of being free to experience and express with another that which he had previously kept hidden. If successful, something new would have happened: he would have broken his old pattern of avoidance; of isolating himself and of saying nothing.

This would by no means be a simple process, because he would bring with him into the therapy room his deeply rooted patterns of avoidance. Apart from creating a climate of respect and engaged attention I would actively try to encourage him to take his own feelings seriously; for example by helping him to verbalize them and if possible to intensify them. That could be done most easily with his dreams, visions and other emotionally laden images from the present and the past. I would, for instance, try to facilitate him in focusing on images from his youth (perhaps of his father and mother) that occurred to him continuously. I would try the same process in regard to the preachers, for whom Hans frequently had very strong bodily feelings of aversion. 'What does this aversion signify?' I would continually ask. The therapeutic aim of this activity would be to make him aware of his bodily felt-experiences and in this way to increase his possibilities to choose.

In this context I would consider it my task to confront Hans with his conflicted feelings. As he himself struggled and doubted for many years, we might well anticipate that this could be a fruitful therapeutic avenue. I would certainly explore with him his feelings towards his wife and ask him whether he realized how much she suffered. And if this turned out to be ineffective, I would express my surprise at him not being aware of the degree to which he caused harm to her and his children. I would do this, of course, without losing my respect and empathic understanding. This is certainly one of the most difficult tasks of the person-centered therapist: to act in congruence with the client in an attitude of empathy, honesty and respect, not personal prejudice.

I might, so far, have given the impression that I would run the risk of trying to change the client in what I consider to be the 'right' direction too quickly—to push too hard. Nothing could be further from the truth. I am well aware that the therapy could be successful only if I were to follow Hans step by step, stay close to him, and not too far ahead. But, from this basic attitude, I would nevertheless confront him at the right moment instead of adopting an attitude of waiting to let things take their course.

I would also consider the possibility of relationship therapy with Hans and his wife and, if they were really willing to take this step, I'm sure this could be very helpful. After all, it is evident that they love each other from the bottom of their hearts. Inwardly, Hans is torn between his love for her and his desire for salvation. She, on her part, continually tries to address and confront him. These could become fruitful relation therapy sessions. Their younger son too could participate in these sessions instead of being completely alone with his problems. The same is true for the eldest son, though for different reasons. These therapeutic actions should of course be taken in the right sequence and within reason.

Considering all this, we should be aware that it is essential for person-centered therapy that the course of events is not fixed beforehand. We may, of course, plan our therapy, formulate goals and intend to use certain interventions. But the process is, and should be, unpredictable in principle and this is precisely the power and attraction of person-centered therapy—that the unexpected determines the course the therapy takes. A person-centered therapist is pre-eminently able to operate flexibly, openly, and to explore everything that occurs in the therapy room. What is more, he or she is able to do so creatively and inventively. In this sense, I can imagine that sooner or later I would start talking to Hans about his particular form of Christian faith. I have no idea, though, how precisely such an interview would go—but I would certainly not avoid it. This does not mean that I would try to convince him to exchange his faith for mine. What it does mean is that I, as a person-centered therapist, would talk with him and try to help him with the problems he has with his life's meaning. In the ideal scenario this would imply that his religious experiences could be disconnected from his neurotic problems. It could well lead to the discovery of another, more healthy, way of religious or spiritual experiencing. This would be a very satisfactory conclusion. The healthy core of his religious obsession could combine with his natural drive, enabling him to lead an enjoyable earthly life. This would be of enormous benefit not only to himself but also to his wife and children.

CONCLUSION

We will never know whether psychotherapy would have been of any use to Hans Sievez. Generally speaking, the question is whether it is possible for somebody with Hans' background to break out of his behavioral patterns and way of being. If at all possible, this would only to a very modest degree be dependent on the therapy and therapist. The capacity of the client would be the crucial factor in this. In the life of Hans Sievez a struggle for life or death is going on between the healthy and the dark forces within him. Nevertheless, therapy can, as modest as its role in this grand drama is, make a crucial difference. And this very difference could bring enormous consequences for Hans and his family. In that sense, we should never underestimate the importance of our work.

The case of Hans Sievez teaches some important lessons for those of us working with clients with religious or spiritual issues. The first is that religious indoctrination, especially the fundamentalistic variety, can be very destructive. What is conspicuous in this is its measure of repetition: the brainwashing takes place from one generation to the other. The case of Hans Sievez demonstrates that this form of conditioning is very hard to overcome. This seems to be independent of the specific form of religion. What is crucial is the degree of fundamentalism involved. This is not to say that religion is destructive per se. This is neither true for religious nor spiritual experiences. On the contrary, the spiritual might well help a person to turn an existential crisis into something positive in his life. This could have been the case for Hans Sievez if he had experienced a healthy spirituality instead of a morbid one. In that case, even those religious visions, which in fact changed his life, could have been helpful for him to find his meaning of life. For the person-centered therapist this might well be a challenge, as the case of Hans Sievez demonstrates. As the representative of a modern system of meaning (van Kalmthout, 2004), there is the dichotomy between two completely different world-views. The challenge, then, is to confront and talk through without losing respect and empathic understanding. The latter, as difficult as this may be, is something we rightly demand from a person-centered therapist.

REFERENCES

Rogers, CR (1980) Ellen West—and loneliness. In CR Rogers *A Way of Being* (pp. 164–80). Boston: Houghton Mifflin Company.

Siebelink, J (2005) *Knielen op een bed violen*. Amsterdam: De Bezige Bij.

Van Kalmthout, M (1997) *Persoonsgerichte psychotherapie*. Utrecht: de Tijdstroom.

Van Kalmthout, M (2002) The farther reaches of person-centered psychotherapy. In J Watson, R Goldman and M Warner (eds) *Client-Centered and Experiential Psychotherapy in the 21st Century: Advances in theory, research and practice* (pp. 127–43). Ross-on-Wye: PCCS Books.

Van Kalmthout, M (2004) Person-centered therapy as a modern system of meaning. *Person-Centered and Experiential Psychotherapies, 3*, 192–206.

Van Kalmthout, M (2005) *Psychotherapie en de zin van het bestaan*. Utrecht: de Tijdstroom.

Van Kalmthout, M (2006) Person-centred psychotherapy as a spiritual discipline. In J Moore and C Purton (eds) *Spirituality and Counselling: Experiential and theoretical perspectives* (pp. 155–68). Ross-on-Wye: PCCS Books.

Van Kalmthout, M (2007) Herhaling van de geschiedenis. Een beschouwing over 'Knielen op een bed violen' van Jan Siebelink. *Tijdschrift Cliëntgerichte Psychotherapie, 44*, 47–56.

CHAPTER 11

THE ART OF PSYCHOLOGICAL CONTACT: THE PSYCHOTHERAPY OF A MENTALLY RETARDED PSYCHOTIC CLIENT[1, 2]

BARBARA KRIETEMEYER AND GARRY PROUTY

INTRODUCTION: GARRY PROUTY

According to Misiak and Sexton (1973: 11), when Abraham Maslow prepared the first general outline of humanistic psychology in 1954 he described it as the scientific study of creativity, love, higher values, autonomy, growth, self-actualization and basic need gratification. Although invaluable as a greatly needed alternative to then-contemporary approaches of psychoanalysis and behaviorism, such a *zeitgeist* seemed not conducive to the study of more severely regressed and institutionalized populations such as individuals with mental retardation, senile dementias or psychoses. This paper presents a therapeutic case history concerning the application of humanistic concepts to a mentally retarded, psychotic client in an institutional setting.

PSYCHOLOGICAL CONTACT

Carl Rogers asserts that the first condition of a therapeutic relationship is psychological contact. He describes this in the following way: 'All that is intended by this first condition is to specify that the two people are to some degree in contact, that each makes some perceived difference in the experiential field of the other' (Rogers, 1957: 96). Prouty (1990) critiques Rogers' description by suggesting that it lacks therapeutic technique or operational constructs. In essence, Rogers did not describe how to develop psychological contact when it is absent; neither did he know how to measure it.

Pre-Therapy as a theory of psychological contact (Prouty, 1994; Prouty, Van Werde and Pörtner, 1998) was developed within the context of treating mentally retarded or psychotic populations (Prouty, 1976, 2001a; Prouty and Cronwall, 1990; Van Werde, 1990; Peters, 1999). The theory of Pre-Therapy is described in three segments: (1) Contact Reflections, (2) Contact Functions, and (3) Contact Behaviors. Contact Reflections refer to the actual work of the therapist; Contact Functions refer to the

---

1. This chapter was first published in *Person-Centered and Experiential Psychotherapies 2*, Autumn, 2003, 151–61.
2. The phrase 'mentally retarded' is the normal language in the USA for this phenomenon. In the UK the same phrase might well be considered inappropriate these days. We remain with the authors' usage (eds).

internal process within the client; and Contact Behaviors refer to emergent behavioral change that can be measured. Complete research, theoretical and philosophical descriptions are available (de Vre, 1992; Dinacci, 1997; Prouty, 1998, 2002, 2003). Numerous practice descriptions are also available (Prouty, 2001b). These articles describe the application of Contact Reflections with diverse populations. The Contact Reflections are: Situational contact, Facial contact, Body contact, Word-for-Word contact, and the Reiterative principle (re-contact).

CONTACT REFLECTIONS

Situational contact
These reflections refer to the therapist following the client's attending to the situation, environment or milieu. An example would be, 'John is looking out the window'. This assists in strengthening or developing *reality contact.*

Facial contact
These reflections are focused toward the pre-expressive feeling in the face. An example is, 'You look sad'. This facilitates *affective contact* within the client.

Word-for-word contact
This style of reflection refers to *communicative contact* with a client who is incoherent. A client may express 'tree' (unintelligible) 'ring' (unintelligible) 'water'. Because this is not understandable, the therapist would reflect word for word, 'tree', 'ring', 'water', even though there is no logic connecting these words.

Body contact
Body reflecting can be illustrated by, 'Your arm is in the air', or 'You are sitting stiffly'. Another variation is for the therapist to use their own body for non-verbal reflections. This assists in the development of body ego (the sense of being 'in' one's body). This is particularly useful for catatonic posturing.

Reiterative contact
This refers to the principle of *re-contact.* There are two forms of reiteration—short-term and long-term. Short-term reiteration is characterized by immediacy. For example, a psychotic girl kept touching her forehead. The therapist kept reflecting this continuously. Finally, the girl said, 'Hurting'. This was then verbally processed into the loss through death of her grandmother, who used to comfort her. An example of long-term reiteration would be the therapist referring to an earlier reflection: 'Last week you pointed to your tummy'. The client responded by a process that led to a discussion of her real pregnancy and traumatic abortion.

These five reflections are extraordinarily literal and concrete. This concreteness is more facilitating of contact in the examples given. This paper illustrates these traditional Pre-Therapy expressions of contact, as well as the more artful forms of contact found in the twenty-five-month therapeutic work of Barbara Krietemeyer with a psychotic, mentally retarded woman. A somewhat different and earlier version of this case was presented in Pörtner (1996).

CASE STUDY: LAURA (BY BARBARA KRIETEMEYER)

This case report is from my experience with a severely handicapped woman in our residential facility. Communication on a pre-expressive, pre-verbal level proved to be an important way to get into contact with her.

Laura, 37, was severely mentally handicapped. At the time I met her, she was going through a period of serious crisis and despair. She quite often screamed and hit her head against the wall; she urinated, defecated and vomited in any setting. Most of the time she lay on her bed undressed. For the last few years, especially since a long-time staff member had left, Laura's condition had become increasingly worse; she refused even the simplest everyday routine, immediately got aggressive, tore up her clothes, threw things around the room, pulled the staff's hair or even tried to bite them in the head. She did the same with her fellow inmates, so that it became impossible to let her be with them. In order to protect her, as well as the others, she quite often had to be tied to her bed and had later been transferred to a very small and cramped single room. In order to maintain some contact with the group, the door had been replaced by a bar with a curtain. Laura became increasingly desperate and emotionally isolated. Only rarely was it possible to get her out of this desperate condition and this was stressful for everybody involved. Laura could not bear contact with others, which, however, she desperately needed. Over time, the space of her internal as well as her external world had become intolerably narrow. The staff felt as if 'Nothing is possible anymore'. They were at their wits' end.

I took Laura over from a colleague who, within a special education program, had taken her for walks five times a week. I started with high ambitions, but was immediately and harshly confronted with reality. As I opened the door, Laura first drew back, then moved straight forward and attacked me. She fought and did not allow me to come near her. Once in a while, I managed to get her dressed and to take her a few steps out of the apartment, but soon she protested and drew me back. Sometimes she tore her clothes to pieces, tried to attack me or whoever happened to be in the way. She wanted to go out, then immediately go in again; she screamed, rushed out again, and finally— desperate—withdrew to her bed. I felt helpless in the face of these fierce manifestations of her will, for which there was no solution in any direction. It remained this way for quite a while. Laura was miserable, I was helpless; both of us were scared of each other— I of her attacks, she of my being a stranger to her.

Finally, I realized that I had to give her more time and space, and to allow her more distance. This was what she really needed: more space to live. This was a cue and a new beginning. I had to find a different way to communicate with her, different from what had been tried before and what I had previously adopted (going into her room and expecting something from her).

127

So I sat down in front of Laura's door. And for a long time I just sat there—on the edge between her world and the world of the group. (*Prouty comments: This is an example of developing a contact boundary between therapist and client.*) This seemed to surprise Laura; I could feel her curious and tense anticipation of what would happen next.

She was lying in her bed. We could not see each other, but were intensely aware of each other's physical presence. (*This awareness of each other was the first step in our developing psychological contact.*) I just sat there in silence. Slowly, I began to perceive what happened around this area. I heard the voices of other inmates and staff members; I was aware of their cheerfulness when they had coffee together; I heard steps coming nearer, and so on. I was also aware of Laura's reactions to what was going on. When she heard the others laugh, she hit her head against the wall; or she jumped abruptly out of bed when a member of staff approached the door. I got the impression that she was also very much aware of how I was present; if I was really with her, or if my attention had diminished. (*This shows the development of a contact rhythm.*) More and more I learned to perceive things in her way and from her perspective; through ears, body, and temperature sense. Instinctively, I began to structure the environment along the same lines as she did and to sort out what was going on in the next room. It was a fascinating experience that I let myself in for completely; and that brought me somewhat nearer to Laura's world. For the first time, a space had been created where we could sense and approach each other, and where contact could slowly develop. (*The therapist empathically understands the structure of the client's experiencing as a condition of a shared world.*)

After two or three weeks, Laura now and then came to the door and stayed there on her knees for a moment, from time to time throwing a quick look at me (*contact*). Then again she withdrew and buried herself deep under the blankets. In this way she went back and forth between bed and door (*contact rhythm*) and presented me with a whole range of expressions; screaming, crying, hitting her head on the floor, listening, waiting, urinating, defecating. She started to rumple her bed and move the mattress on the floor. I saw this as a sign that within her something had started to move.

Laura sometimes clicked her tongue or knocked with her fingers on the walls and door. (*Client expresses her mode of contact with reality.*) I then brought with me some things we could play with. Laura pricked up her ears at the clicking of marbles or at the soft sounds of the tambourine. From time to time I rolled the marbles into her room. Laura looked at them interestedly and then threw them out again. (*Psychological contact has been established.*) She started to respond to my beating the drum by beating the floor with her fingers, distinctly taking up my rhythm. Sometimes an intense interplay developed, a mutual calling and answering. These were exciting (and for Laura also amusing) moments of contact with each other.

What at first had seemed to be just a stopgap (to sit at the doorstep and silently allow contact and proximity) turned out to be a real chance for progress. Laura could herself measure out this contact, and could withdraw or come closer as it suited her (*primitive actualization*) and as far as she could bear it. Also, I could change my sitting position and observe how Laura reacted to that. Two or three months later a situation arose that brought me to continue to stick with my position at the door: Laura's condition became dramatically worse. (*This is often the case when dealing with intense affective experiencing.*) Again and again she hit her head on the floor, screamed and cried. Then, slowly, the aggressions against herself turned into desperate crying and sobbing. It was as if her whole misery and shock would burst out once more. However, at the end of the sessions she usually calmed down. During this period of time, Laura intensely lived through her fear, her anxiety and her lack of foundation. I could do nothing but be with her, acknowledge her emotions and empathically endure them with her. Once, deeply touched by her crying, I reflected spontaneously in a very soft voice, 'You feel so miserable, you are so sad' (*situational reflection*). The effect was incredible; I had reached her, though till then she had not seemed to respond to language.

As time went by, the crying diminished and Laura began to feel considerably better. Her moods still fluctuated, but on the whole she seemed happier now and less desperate. Staff members observed that in daily life Laura's spirits were now on a different level. A next step lay ahead: to open the door of her room. As I had expected, this once more led to her throwing flowerpots and other things around. The sessions became a zigzag path; out in the living room, throwing chairs around the room, back to bed again, screaming, coming out again, etc. I tried to help Laura to handle at least short sequences without aggression, and then to slowly extend these periods. It turned out to be helpful to do this along with familiar activities like getting dressed, sitting at the table and having coffee. At the beginning, for Laura, this was just a matter of a few seconds. For a very short time, with my presence and body contact, I could offer her some support. Sitting next to her and holding her hand, I reflected the situation (*situational reflections*), such as, 'Laura is drinking coffee', 'Laura is sitting at the table'.

It was extremely difficult to give Laura enough space for her actions, and also to set limits for her when the chaos within her became overwhelming. Then, I had to bring her back to her room, close the door, and keep contact there. It was a continuous shuttle between these two poles where I had to adjust to her abrupt changes. She led the way (*non-directivity*). It was different every day. I followed her with a goal in my mind, but had to make enormous sidesteps in all directions. Laura herself often wanted much more than she could carry through so I had to be aware of her limits and to re-establish them if necessary. To continuously maintain this balance was, at that time, the main issue of my working with her.

After a while the staff observed that Laura's tolerance for being more in contact increased. In her cramped conditions every inch counted: Laura would wait a little after the door was unlocked: a meaningful moment, and soon she spontaneously opened the door to go to the bathroom by herself. Such tiny opportunities for self-determination and use of her own power enormously reinforced Laura's self-esteem. She obviously enjoyed these activities. Despite her still rather disgraceful life conditions, these were small qualitative steps to which Laura answered with a smile. Encouraged by these first steps the staff looked for niches in the daily routine in which Laura could regain her abilities to do things and to express herself. This required a new attitude towards Laura: not to reach out to her, but to wait until she herself took the initiative or picked up an impulse. Moreover, we had to handle her strong will and her impatience. She screamed when she had to wait a few moments for her clothes in getting dressed. It then helped to ask her where the clothes could possibly be. I started to look around for them and encouraged her to help me. This quite often worked.

At the beginning I had never imagined that Laura would be open to verbal responses. Verbally reflecting her actions obviously helped her to better recognize her competencies and her personal power. This showed in the energy with which she opened a door or stamped her feet when walking. Short sentences like, 'Laura opens the door', and sharing her pleasure in doing so, seemed to anchor her perception more deeply in her experiencing. The word 'Wait', for example, was particularly meaningful because it was so difficult for her to endure even a short moment of waiting, for instance for a staff member to bring her coffee. Therefore I consciously waited with her and said, 'Laura has to wait. K went to get the coffee,' (*situational reflections*) and so on. Laura obviously learned to connect the attitude with the word and to internalize it. In her relations with the staff, Laura became more open to language and could deal increasingly well with various situations in everyday life.

Laura now extended her radius to the park. She explored spaces and pulled me single-mindedly to where she wanted to go. From now on, verbally reflecting her intentions and her experiencing of reality became a crucial part of my working with her. Over and over again I could observe how this helped Laura to become more concise and self-confident in her ways of expressing herself. So when we left the apartment, she sometimes hummed her favorite song, 'Muss i denn, muss i denn zum Städtele hinaus'— and I very happily joined in.

So far the staff had always led Laura by the hand. Even at meals she often needed this as a support as well as to prevent her aggression. Now, when she wanted something on our way, she pulled me by the hand, screaming. I started now and then to free myself from her grip and to push her hand gently away saying, 'Show me what you want. Where do you want to go?' And she actually started to walk ahead. It did not always work, especially when she was in an unstable, fragile condition and needed my hand for support. But it became increasingly possible. So I took advantage of the favorable periods to try out new steps, whereas in other periods I considerably lowered my ambitions.

After many weeks, a staff member told me that on walks Laura now often refused to give her hand because she obviously wanted to walk ahead by herself. This beautifully proved that Laura was able to transfer experiences from our sessions to other situations and people, and showed that she was growing.

I now started to take Laura to a gym and playroom regularly where I intended to spend part of our time in a playful way simulating interactions. This was the first time she had ventured beyond her own room and those rooms needed for daily care. Here too, she was the one who led the direction. At first, we could stay only very briefly, then she withdrew to the bathroom or started to undress or lie down on the rocking bed, which soon became her favorite place for peace and retreat. Again, I offered her sounds as a bridge and as a symbol of contact from me to her: humming and tambourine sounds (*reiterative reflections*). Laura listened carefully. A caring closeness developed, which she enjoyed. Sometimes she hummed a song to herself. Sometimes I put a tambourine next to her or held it out to her, and very shyly she tried to make sounds. She greatly enjoyed the resonance of the sounds her actions provoked—they were as an echo of her.

I would like to make a few remarks about how I see music as a 'language of the soul'. In addition to the stimulating experiences these activities provide, I see music as a mirror of the inner world, of moods and feelings, where a person may rediscover in the sound something of herself—even if in only a vague and diffused way, as was the case with Laura. But even the most primitive discoveries with sounds are a beginning and, in my opinion, more than a sensual stimulation. It is the experience: 'This is how what I do sounds, this is how I sound' (*self-sense*).

Laura became stronger psychologically in her confrontations. These no longer basically indicated that she could not cope with a situation, but more and more turned into a struggle for self-assertion that she joyfully acted out. For me it was harder this way, but for Laura it was an important threshold. She could now more fully enjoy her strength on a more solid ground. Sometimes, when she was definitely annoyed and angry, I responded to her anger: 'Laura is shouting, Laura is annoyed' (*situational reflections*), and then led her to the big drums. I encouraged her to scold, together with me, on the drums. She did so by fiercely beating the drum with her index finger, thus intensively experiencing her anger. I could not help smiling when a staff member told me later that Laura now, from time to time, got really angry and drummed so fiercely on the table that she made the coffee cups rattle.

These great moments were like real flashes which, now and then, illuminated Laura's potential. However, the possibility of stimulating anything strongly depended on her condition at that moment. What was possible today could be impossible tomorrow. Her psychological structure, to a certain extent, remained unstable and fragile. Also, no other solution of her living situation came into view. And yet, some qualitative changes emerged: Laura could be cheerful again, she had rediscovered her smile and her giggle, and the self-aggression considerably diminished. Sometimes the staff could now take her on a walk with the group. Laura could stand it better to be with others; she was able to have coffee or dinner with them, and it became possible to take her to the playground. She participated more actively in the daily routine; she helped get herself dressed and washed her own hands; in the morning she went to the toilet without being controlled, and by herself she cleared the dishes to the kitchen.

The staff member who was closest to her shared her impression: before, Laura had existed only by the external structure we offered her. Now she discovered internal stability, some self-esteem and a grounding she had not known before. In the two years I worked with Laura, regaining this grounding was a crucial step for her growing—even if from time to time it diminished or broke. To this day (two and a half years later) she has never reached crisis stage again.

So much for my work with Laura. I have described my way of proceeding as it developed in working with her: searching for new ways, trying things out, being confronted again and again with doubts, limits and questions. On the basis of client-centered and play therapy, but also with systemic views in my 'hand baggage', I tried out whatever Laura offered or admitted, and whatever helped to approach her.

131

CONCLUSION: BARBARA KRIETEMEYER

Only by looking back can I describe my work under the aspect of Pre-Therapy methods. I will try to summarize the most important elements.

To begin with, the offer of a therapeutic relationship happened, basically, in a pre-verbal, pre-symbolic space. I had to relate to the structure of Laura's inner world and, at the beginning, to do so without verbal language. There are two main points I want to stress. First, shared perception: we started to have contact as soon as I tried to understand Laura's perception by perceiving things, as much as possible, through the same senses as she did. This opened a door for me into her experiencing.

The second point is shared experiences and feelings: I began to empathically perceive and sense Laura's feelings and moods, her needs and anxieties, her despair and anger, her inner chaos, and so on. I believe that to experience with her, be with her and bear with her was the essential thing. Let me use a musical image to describe it: resonance. Contact emerges when I am able to create resonance. There is a point where both vibrations meet and create something in common. We can, in a very concrete way, experience resonance in relationships. In therapy, I must be able to resonate in order to reach the other person. I believe that severely handicapped people are especially sensitive to this kind of communication. Sometimes it becomes a tightrope walk: there is always the possibility of projections and misunderstandings. At some points a 'melting together' may arise and limits may become blurred. But at the same time, in all this, there is a chance; to experience how, in this encounter, isolation can be abolished. Later on, when Laura became more open for words, verbal reflections began to take an important place. As she did not talk, I tried to reflect as much as possible what she expressed and what she did, especially:

- Situational Reflections (*reflection of environmental interactions*)
- Body Reflections (*reflection of bodily expression*)
- Facial Reflections (*reflection of not-yet-verbalized feeling in the face*).

This obviously helped Laura to become more conscious and more present in her own ways of expressing herself. She began to enjoy that. Thus, the verbal reflections had also encouraged her emotional life.

At some points, beyond mere contact reflections, I also verbalized Laura's feelings and intentions. I do not know if these more abstract notions did reach her. But at least she could understand the tune that accompanied them. I also used the sounds of my voice and the tambourines as a bridge to Laura, as a means of communicative contact. Music, in a unique way, links the different aspects of contact; communication and symbolization of experiences and emotions.

To sum up, I can say that I consider Pre-Therapy ways of communication to be relevant when pre-verbal relational experience is impaired or not sufficiently developed. It is important to use these specific qualities of relation as a conscious therapeutic attitude. To offer this kind of relation is, in my experience, not just a granted basic attitude but in itself an effective therapeutic factor.

FURTHER DISCUSSION: GARRY PROUTY

This case history illustrates the application of *psychological contact* with a very regressed, mentally retarded and psychotic client. Besides applying the traditional Situational, Facial, Bodily, Word-for-Word and Reiterative reflections, the therapist creatively used other aspects of psychological contact. The first technique, that of 'entering' the *structure of what* the client was experiencing, was similar to the work of Prouty (1986) in reflecting the structure of the hallucination. The difference is Krietemeyer's application to realistic experience, as compared to hallucinatory experience. The second technique was discovering the client's *mode of contact*. In this case it was sound and music. This enabled the therapist to have the opportunity to access the client's *path to reality*. The next issue, that of *contact rhythm*, is significant. Contact moves to and fro between persons. It is important to be aware of this ebb and flow as process, and to be accepting of it rather than trying to push for steady contact. As a result of accepting the ebb and flow, a more intense expression of emotion appeared. This case history also reveals the extremely concrete nature of the therapist's responses. The case study raises the possibility that psychological contact can be described, in Buber's (1964: 547) words as the art of 'pointing to the concrete'.

REFERENCES

Buber, M (1964) Phenomenological analysis of existence versus pointing to the concrete. In M Friedman (ed) *The Worlds of Existentialism: A critical reader.* New York: Random House.

Dinacci, A (1997) Ricerca sperimentale sul trattamento psicologico dei pazienti schizofrenici con la pre-therapia di Dr. G Prouty. *Psicologia della persona, II,* 4, 7–16.

De Vre, R (1992) *Prouty's Pre-Therapie.* Rijksuniversiteit Eindverhandeling Licentiaat Psychologie, Gent (Dept. of Psychology, University of Ghent, Belgium).

Misiak, H and Sexton, V (1973) *Phenomenological, Existential and Humanistic Psychologies: A historical survey.* New York: Grune and Stratton.

Peters, H (1999) Pre-Therapy: An approach to mentally handicapped people. *Journal of Humanistic Psychology, 39,* 4, 8–29.

Pörtner, M (1996) A hopeless case. In *Trust and Understanding: The person-centred approach to everyday care for people with special needs* (pp. 105–13). Ross-on-Wye: PCCS Books.

Prouty, G (1976) Pre-Therapy: A method of treating pre-expressive psychotic and retarded clients. *Psychotherapy: Theory, research and practice, 13,* 290–4.

Prouty, G (1986) The pre-symbolic structure and therapeutic transformations of hallucinations. In M Wolpin, J Shore and L Krueger (eds) *Imagery, Vol. 4* (pp. 99–106). New York: Plenum Press.

Prouty, G (1990) Pre-Therapy: A theoretical evolution in the person-centered/experiential psychotherapy of schizophrenia and retardation. In G Lietaer, J Rombauts and R Van Balen (eds) *Client-Centered and Experiential Psychotherapy in the Nineties* (pp. 645–58). Leuven: Leuven University Press.

Prouty, G (1994) *Theoretical Evolutions in Person-Centered/Experiential Therapy: Applications to schizophrenic and retarded psychoses.* Westport, CT: Praeger (Greenwood).

Prouty, G (1998) Pre-Therapy and the pre-expressive self. *Person-Centred Practice, 6*, 80–8.

Prouty, G (2001a) Pre-Therapy: A treatment method for people with mental retardation who are also psychotic. In A Dosen and K Day (eds) *Treating Mental Illness and Behavior Disorders in Children and Adults with Mental Retardation* (pp. 155–66). Washington, DC: American Psychiatric Press.

Prouty, G (2001b) The practice of Pre-Therapy. *Journal of Contemporary Psychotherapy, 31*, 31–40.

Prouty, G (2002) Humanistic psychotherapy for people with schizophrenia. In D Cain and J Seeman (eds) *Humanistic Psychotherapies: Handbook of research and practice* (pp. 579–601). Washington, DC: American Psychological Association.

Prouty, G (2003) Prä-Therapie: Eine Einführung zur Philosophie und Theorie. In W Keil and G Stumm (eds) Die vielen Gesichter der Personzentrierten Psychotherapie (pp. 499–512). Vienna: Springer.

Prouty, G and Cronwall, M (1990) Psychotherapeutic approaches in the treatment of depression in mentally retarded adults. In A Dosen and F Menaolascino (eds) *Depression in Mentally Retarded Children and Adults* (pp. 281–93). Leiden, Netherlands: Logan Publications.

Prouty, G, Van Werde, D and Pörtner, M (1998) *Prä-Therapie.* Stuttgart: Klett-Cotta.

Prouty, G, Van Werde, D and Pörtner, M (2002) *Pre-Therapy: Reaching contact-impaired clients.* Ross-on-Wye: PCCS Books.

Rogers, CR (1957) The necessary and sufficient conditions of therapeutic personality change. *Journal of Consulting Psychology, 21*, 95–105.

Van Werde, D (1990) Psychotherapy with a retarded, schizo-affective woman: An application of Prouty's Pre-Therapy. In A Dosen, A Van Gennep and G Zwanikken (eds) *Treatment of Mental Illness and Behavioral Disorder in the Mentally Retarded* (pp. 469–77). Proceedings of the International Congress, Amsterdam. Leiden: Logan Publications.

CHAPTER 12

THE FALLING MAN: PRE-THERAPY APPLIED TO SOMATIC HALLUCINATING[1]

DION VAN WERDE

4. Because wisdom will not enter into a soul that deviseth evil, Nor dwell in a body that is held in pledge by sin.

5. For a holy spirit of discipline will flee deceit, And will start away from thoughts that are without understanding, And will be put to confusion when unrighteousness hath come in.

6. For wisdom is a spirit that loveth man, And she will not hold a blasphemer guiltless for his lips; Because God beareth witness of his reins, And is a true overseer of his heart, And a hearer of his tongue.

Book of Wisdom (Ch. 1, vv. 4–6)

This chapter describes a piece of therapy undertaken in a multidisciplinary residential psychiatric setting. It involved working with a man 'Henry' who has the utmost incongruence between himself and the experiencing of his body. During treatment, and especially with the help of individual sessions based on Pre-Therapy, the client literally achieved a new balance, with the result that he no longer insisted on vehemently and physically correcting his hallucinatory body problems. He mastered the problematic relationship with his body sufficiently to leave the hospital and to move to vocational training and a paid job.

The chapter assumes a certain familiarity with Pre-Therapy as described by Prouty (1976, 1990, 1994) and Van Werde (1994, 1998) (see also Prouty, Van Werde and Pörtner, 2002) and, specifically, the use of contact reflections: that is, forms of reflections of concrete client behaviour by which the therapist makes contact with the client, and which are designed to establish and enhance the client's contact functions. Contact reflections take five forms (originally identified by Prouty, 1976): Situational, Facial, Body, Word-for-Word and Reiterative.

---

1. This chapter was originally published in *Person-Centred Practice 10,* Autumn, 2002, 101–7.

THE CLIENT

The client, Henry, a man of average intelligence and in his early twenties, was an in-patient in our psychiatric hospital for approximately one year. Six years earlier, following a *fugue* (a sudden flight from home) and his subsequent return, Henry's parents had taken him to a psychiatrist. He was always bad tempered, and he and his parents quarrelled endlessly. At the time of the initial referral, he had just come back from a Scouts' camp, exhausted from a series of late nights with an average of only two hours sleep: 'It was hot there and I wanted to feel myself awake so badly' was his comment. He was then referred to a psychiatric hospital. He went home after seven weeks with a prescription for a maintenance dose of neuroleptic drugs (Melleril® 100 mg a day).

The fights at home stopped and the family was relatively satisfied. The parents decided to take him out of school and have him start as an assistant in a friend's grocery store. Gradually, Henry became interested in the Bible. He clearly prayed more than before. Working and studying lost importance for him. He felt himself becoming holy: 'I looked radiant. I often stood in front of the mirror and found myself beautiful'. At the same time, he had thoughts compelling him to injure other people: to 'hit them in the face'. The client had to discipline himself not to give in to these thoughts: 'They were all thoughts that made me unhappy and gave me a headache. I was always busy with them'.

This situation worsened and a year later the client became convinced that he had to exorcise the Devil to let God enter:

> There are good things in myself but they can't come out. My heart is like a stone, my body needs to be refreshed. The Holy Spirit lives in my abdomen, I need to let God come in from above, to have him make contact with the Spirit and expel the Devil out of my body. I let everything come to my heart. I must proclaim my guilt and sweat water and blood, one hundred per cent intense.

From that time on, the client started literally to practise what he said. He developed a way of falling and screaming that was designed to put an end to his sinful life. The way he experienced his body was very bizarre. He had the idea that his organs had changed places. Thus, he thought that his shoulders had narrowed and that the part between his shoulders had descended in the direction of his belly and pubic region. The falling was meant to shock his body in such a way that his organs returned to where they belonged. He jumped in the air and threw himself on his knees to the floor. This was accompanied by a gruesome noise, especially because he felt that while falling he must confess all his sins. Once he had been admitted to our ward (aged twenty-one), we heard this repeated falling, together with a hardly comprehensible recitation of sins. This falling and screaming put the whole ward under tremendous strain.

THE THEORY

We would describe the problem as one of somatic hallucinating involving a delusional interpretation of a bizarre bodily perception. When somebody is suffering psychosis (in this case a psychosis concerning the body) contact is lost and psychosomatic balance is disturbed. Functioning, both psychological and factual, is out of personal control and is in conflict with collective expectations, rules, norms and so on. On top of this the person is afraid of holding still, of looking at experiences that 'pop up' and tend to take over, since these are so powerful and overwhelming. This leads to alienation, stress and isolation.

The concept of treatment, especially from the perspective of Pre-Therapy, is to accompany the person in their search for contact. The application of Pre-Therapy to a ward milieu is extensively described in Prouty, Van Werde and Pörtner (2002). During the treatment, in the context of the psychiatric ward, the person is individually helped to restore their balance, to break the psychotic isolation, and to build up healthy functioning. Since we work in an institution, and are in charge of twenty-four patients, we have to confront the client continuously with the demands on him or her because there is more than one single individual and they do not function in a vacuum. There are the realities of the fellow patients, the house-rules, the timetables, and so on. Part of our task—our mission—is to find a way to bridge the patients' individual needs and the structural limitations of an institution and a regime. As to individual needs, we make sure that we stay attuned to the emotional world of the people we work with in order to facilitate psychotherapeutic process if at all possible. At the same time, we have no difficulty in actively integrating reality elements into our work. However, we are aware that, in the last instance, it is the client who decides what should be done and, taking everything into account, what is best for him or her.

We try to stay with whatever presents itself, even when, for ourselves, the things that occur are new and, at first sight, incomprehensible. Staff also need regular support to be able to live this phenomenological attitude continuously, to tolerate all the bizarre behaviours, and to continue to trust experiential processes (Deleu and Van Werde, 1998). Experiencing this attitude enables the patient to build up their strength from within and eventually start the psychotherapeutic process (hence 'Pre-Therapy'); he is reconnecting with parts of his functioning that have become alien even to him.

What follows is a brief description of the therapy of Henry (the 'falling man') over approximately one year of in-patient treatment.

THE THERAPY

Most of the time and in almost every social situation, 'the falling man' could act normally, albeit on a superficial level. He even over-achieved in being courteous and helpful. However, especially when alone, he could lose himself easily and plunge into his own swamps of bizarre pre-expressive functioning. At the behest of his family, almost nobody knew of his admission to the hospital: it was a well-kept secret. This situation fortified his psychological isolation.

Once he had arrived on our ward, the problem of ensuring ward structure and keeping up house-rules very soon conflicted with periods of this client's pre-expressive functioning. His dangerous behaviour necessitated intervention in his process. If we continued to let him do his 'exercises' (as he called them), we would expose other patients to incomprehensible noises of repeated falling and fast-spoken words. This was one of the considerations in limiting his behaviour; another came from our responsibility and concern for his physical safety. Several times he did real damage to himself by falling on the floor. At one point, fluid in his knees needed draining off. Another referral to a general hospital occurred when he lost fluid from his nose (possibly of cerebral origin). Other limits that were set and measures that were taken during his stay included forbidding him to sit in the room of another patient and sing and pray aloud during the night. As far as we were able, the nursing staff and myself tried to stay with his process and, in doing so, to help him to re-contact his own proactive forces. We did this not only by listening to his words and paying attention to his behaviour but also by always consciously trying to capture the facial signs of concurrent affective life and offer it back to him, often by means of Facial Reflections (FRs). Thus, when he came out of his room after the nurses had reminded him that it was time for coffee (Situational Reflections—SRs), they reflected (FR) 'You smile' or 'You look puzzled' (FR) or even 'You look anxious' (FR). Sometimes they went to the toilet or the bathroom to reflect that they had heard him on the corridor or in the bathroom (SR). This was done to be with his falling and screaming in places that he thought private by offering him the realities about noise, sound, volume, etc. They reflected his sitting in front of the television (SR) (that was turned off) and looking like he was daydreaming (FR). They reflected him saying that he had pain in his coccyx (Word-for-Word Reflections) but also his smiling (FR) at the same time. Sometimes these reflections brought him into contact with the reality of his body and even with his life which, until that moment, had been transposed into pre-expressive bizarre behaviour (for instance, pain and smiling). Little by little he contacted his doubts, his shame, his need for reassurance, his fear of the future and so on.

Treatment did not become standardised but stayed tailor-made—but within certain boundaries. Parallel to his self-abuse (falling, exaggerated jogging, binge-eating, staying awake at night to pray, hurting his toes by repetitive exercises to stretch his pelvis), nursing staff talked to him about how to take care of his body, for instance by sitting in the sun to dry out pimples, using a different shampoo to deal with dandruff and so on. In this sense, working on contact in general and working on contact with his body in particular was not reduced to focusing only on the bizarre and the damage done. It stayed as open as possible, thus including positive aspects of attention and care for himself. Other actions undertaken by the nurses included having him draw up his activities for one week and discussing with him the lack of spare moments. They told him about pain as a valuable signal given by the body. They informed him about the dangers of damaging his knees and head. They repeatedly explained to him why he was given medication to sleep and why sleeping is important.

Gradually, through his treatment, an opening up towards other people, reality in general and towards his body, together with a de-freezing of his affective life, became visible. Over the year cracks appeared in the façade of being perfect and without problems. More and more people became aware of his bizarre habit of falling and confessing: first the nurses, then the psychologist (Henry started demonstrating his 'exercises' in his office) and even his fellow patients. When we gave him this reality-information it really shook him up, since this undermined his routine of exercising and disturbed his frozen social balances. Nursing staff also became stricter as to what was allowed and what was not. All this intensified his psychological process. He began to talk about being abused as a child and feeling like a lamb to the slaughter. He felt himself bad and sinful and punished by God. Treatment skill was demonstrated in following the tempo of his process without compromising the ward's structure too much, and without being scared away by his actions. We were able to maintain him on our ward and have him participate in the programme without cutting across his psychological process. Concrete therapeutic progress was made.

A key episode in his treatment arose when the individual psychotherapist no longer tolerated Henry's falling 'exercises' in his office (which at that time was located on the ward itself). Since Henry had opened up and started sharing consciously this hidden aspect of his life, the therapist had not wanted to stop this process. So, after thorough deliberation, the psychotherapist suggested that they work together in a soundproofed room above the hospital gym. They would not be disturbed there nor would they disturb anybody else. The offer to change location was responsive to the reality of life on the ward (in terms of noise and sound) and it acknowledged the necessary limitations of the institution.

The first session above the gym involved a lot of talking and resembled the sessions in the office. Near the end of that particular session, the client himself proposed practising his falling. They agreed that a gym mat would be used to prevent severe physical damage. The next ten minutes were very intense. Henry would stand staring, his legs wide open, stretching his upper body, then proceed to confess his sins whilst falling down flat on the mat, his hands pushing his pelvis up. The therapist used Pre-Therapy reflections intensively to stay with that process. These aimed to help Henry fully contact his experiencing and what he was doing with, and to, his body, thereby shifting his level from pre-expressive to expressive functioning: 'You are standing upright' (Body Reflections—BRs), 'Your face looks pale' (FR), 'You stare' (FR), 'You fall down'(BR), 'I hear you fall down on the mat' (SR), 'You look very concentrated' (FR), 'I hear you call out your sins aloud' (SR), 'You fell again' (BR, Reiterative Reflection—RR), 'Your knuckles are white' (BR), 'You put at lot of pressure on your pelvis' (BR), 'You look at me' (SR), 'We're above the gym' (SR), 'You said you wanted to exercise' (RR), 'It looks like you're in pain' (FR). To the latter Henry replied 'Of course I am in pain! Do you think that it doesn't hurt?' By saying this, he started contacting his feelings. His tempo slowed. Then he wanted to stop the session and, after the therapist had reiterated what had happened, they agreed to meet again some days later.

For the second session, in the same location above the gym, Henry came a few minutes late. He started talking. After a while, he said that falling was not necessary anymore. The therapist was genuinely very surprised and asked the reason for his new position. Henry said that he had just visited the hospital priest; he had confessed all his sins and had been forgiven! This made his continued falling (in order to exclaim all his sins and change his body) redundant. Everything was now OK!

After this, we saw that Henry needed to fall less. He had made a therapeutic shift. A new balance was achieved and this evolution was consolidated. The client moved to a rehabilitation ward and was able to take up employment training. Some months later he started a job and, five years later, he was still working. No crisis intervention or admission has been necessary since. He lived with his parents again without too many difficulties. His GP regularly prescribed a minimal dose of neuroleptic drugs to support his psychological balance. When contacted for follow-up, and to ask permission to publish his case, he told his former psychiatrist that he still occasionally 'exercised', but far less intensely and far less frequently. It had never hindered him in his work. Follow up after ten years showed that, after five years, he had given up independent employment as the pressure had been too great. Together with moving into a sheltered living accommodation, relatively satisfying conditions were set and are still held, to consolidate the balance achieved so arduously: his stress was reduced by stopping the regular job and changing to working on a farm for some days a week on a voluntary basis.

CONCLUSION

As a person-centred team we experience the importance and therapeutic relevance of welcoming and staying with any material that presents itself or that is jointly chosen to look at. The client's experiencing as well as the institutional demands are the continuous touchstones of everything that is undertaken. We learn that the restoration and strengthening of contact are the basic processes and outcomes of our work.

How do we conceptualise the psychotherapeutic process that took place—and what happened to the somatic hallucination? On admission, we saw that Henry's psychological space almost coincided with his experience, as if his organs really had changed position and needed to be restored to their right place again. Connected to this, but on a different level, was his self-awareness as being 'evil' and 'punished'. Falling and confessing his sins would 'forgive' his sins and also, literally, put everything in place again. Social functioning had been impossible; his isolation was almost complete. On the ward, this person, including his problematic experiencing and behaving, was welcomed. Staff also acted normally towards clearly psychotic functioning. By not being absorbed in his 'bodily problem', as he himself obviously was, staff could gradually anchor the man back to reality (see Van Werde, 1998), and bring him into communication.

The hypothesis of Pre-Therapy—that contact and symptomatic functioning are inversely connected—appears plausible and proven. The more Henry engaged in the therapeutic process, the less he needed to block every feeling, every other human being and every bit of 'shared reality' out of his life. Somatic hallucinating no longer dominated his total functioning. It became condensed and dissolved a little into healthy functioning. Generally, he started feeling and acting again with respect for his body, to sense its limits and possibilities.

In the end, the psychotic core was addressed. We saw Henry eagerly starting his exercising. Then, after having really contacted what he was doing, he refrained from plunging into that explosive and dark area of hidden meanings and engraved history. He decided to stop and, in a manner of speaking, accepted the shifted balance. Problematic functioning became less dominating in his life, although not completely resolved. Overall, he felt strong enough to take control of his own life again.

REFERENCES

Deleu, C and Van Werde D (1998) The relevance of a phenomenological attitude when working with psychotic people. In B Thorne and E Lambers (eds) *Person-Centred Therapy: A European perspective* (pp. 206–15). London: Sage.

Prouty, G (1976) Pre-therapy: A method of treating pre-expressive psychotic and retarded patients. *Psychotherapy: Theory, research and practice, 13,* 290–95.

Prouty, G (1990) A theoretical evolution in the person-centered/experiential psychotherapy of schizophrenia and retardation. In G Lietaer, J Rombauts and R Van Balen (eds) *Client-Centered and Experiential Psychotherapy in the Nineties* (pp. 645–85). Leuven: Leuven University Press.

Prouty, G (1994) *Theoretical Evolutions in Person-Centered/Experiential Therapy: Applications to schizophrenic and retarded psychoses.* New York: Praeger.

Prouty, G, Van Werde, D and Pörtner, M (2002) *Pre-Therapy.* Ross-on-Wye: PCCS Books.

Van Werde, D (1994a) An introduction to client-centred pre-therapy. In D Mearns, *Developing Person-Centred Counselling* (pp. 120–4). London: Sage.

Van Werde, D (1994b) Dealing with the possibility of psychotic content in a seemingly congruent communication. In D Mearns, *Developing Person-Centred Counselling* (pp. 125–8). London: Sage.

Van Werde, D (1998) Anchorage as a core concept in working with psychotic people. In B Thorne and E Lambers (eds) *Person-Centred Therapy: A European perspective* (pp. 195–205). London: Sage.

CHAPTER 13

LUKE'S PROCESS: A POSITIVE VIEW OF SCHIZOPHRENIC THOUGHT DISORDER

MARGARET S. WARNER

INTRODUCTION

I have been working for some thirteen years with 'Luke',[1] a client who thinks in the very unusual ways typically labeled as 'schizophrenic thought disorder'.[2] This kind of 'thought disorder' isn't the only kind of symptom that schizophrenic people experience, but it is a very common one, repeatedly described in the literature on schizophrenia since the late nineteenth century. Let me give you an example of this kind of thinking on Luke's part.

One day Luke had lunch with his father and a Catholic priest who was a family friend. The priest lamented the fact that in recent days Catholics were 'going to the dogs'. Luke, who is Catholic, had never considered the possibility that he might be about to become a dog. But, he spent the next weekend carefully scrutinizing dogs he saw in the park to see how they were doing. He decided that they mostly seemed to have smiles on their faces, so he came to the conclusion that turning into a dog might not be such a terrible thing.

Most schools of psychotherapy discourage attending to this sort of 'thought disordered' train of thought for fear of encouraging thinking that is irrational. In most therapeutic orientations, therapists who do listen empathically to such thoughts, do this primarily as a prelude to some other sort of intervention aimed at correcting the person's flawed thinking or behavior. Person-centered therapists—especially those following the work of Garry Prouty[3]—take a very different approach. We suggest that human beings have extremely deep tendencies and desires to make sense of their own experience. And, we believe that, if clients are empathically understood and valued in a genuine way, they are extremely likely to move toward personally meaningful and realistic ways of making sense of their experience. Prouty (Prouty, 1994; Prouty et al., 2002) suggests that empathic responding that stays very close to the person's exact words, gestures, facial expressions and the like is particularly likely to help make psychological contact with clients who are out of normative relation to 'self', 'world' or 'other'.

---

1. Significant names and places are altered in this account to preserve 'Luke's' confidentiality.
2. For a review of the literature on thought disorder, see Warner (2007, in press).
3. See, for example, Prouty (1994) Prouty et al., (2002), Warner (2006) and Rogers et al., (1967).

If you have never tried this, it may seem very counter-intuitive to you. How could sensible conclusions come from these sorts of 'crazy' thoughts? I know that I didn't know *what* to expect when I first started seeing Luke. I had fantasies that he might spin out of control and run out the room screaming or some such. Much of the therapeutic literature suggests that schizophrenic people are unable to use introspective psychotherapies very well.[4] Research finds that schizophrenic clients have particular difficulty making sense of their own feelings and intentions.[5] And schizophrenic clients are seen as having great difficulty handling social interactions, with the result that they often become very socially reclusive.[6]

So, it was an act of pure faith for me to believe that if I just tried to express my understanding of Luke's experience something good would happen. And, as it happens, a number of strikingly good things *have* happened over the years. Psychotic experiences that were so frightening that Luke felt the need to respond in defensive ways have stopped happening almost entirely. (This is not to say that Luke doesn't have psychotic experiences, but the experiences that he does have tend not to be frightening.) He has an increasingly positive sense of himself and confidence that he can make sense of experiences that seem confusing or threatening. Luke used to dress in ways that looked odd, whereas now he dresses in a normative, even distinguished-looking, way. He is still confused about the factual causes of some events in his life but he comes to very sensible and personally grounded understandings of his feelings, intentions and wants. And with this increased confidence he has become strikingly pro-social. He typically writes a number of letters or postcards each week to family or friends and carefully thinks through social interactions and trips that he would like to take part in. And he follows through, contacting people, figuring out logistics and going on social outings that he enjoys.

Luke's life is quite limited compared to that of most non-schizophrenic people and he still processes his experiences in ways that are very different from most people. But after starting therapy as a frightened and often tormented person, he has come to have a life that is grounded, personally satisfying to him, and socially engaged. A few years back Luke noted that he was glad that his life had come together before his father's death and that he was able to have 'some little pride in himself'.

Over time I began to think of Luke's way of thinking as a difficult, but fundamentally positive, way of processing experience one that I am now calling 'metaphact processing'. This is a style of processing that joins more ordinary facts and metaphors[7] into a single

---

4. See Thase and Jindal (2004) for a review of recent research on approaches to therapy with schizophrenia. Karon and VandenBos (1981) on the other hand, have achieved very good outcome results working with a humanistically oriented form of psychotherapy.
5. M Brune (2005) has written an excellent summary of research documenting difficulties that schizophrenic people often have with forming accounts of their own and other people's feelings, intentions, desires and the like.
6. E. Fuller Torrey, MD (1983: 38–44) vividly describes some of the withdrawal experiences of schizophrenic people.
7. I am using the word metaphor in its broad sense here, including those figures of speech that indicate some broad similarity rather than a clearly defined identity. More specific figures of speech such as similes and personification are subsumed in the terms 'metaphor' and 'metaphoric distance' in this chapter.

hybrid form at times when the person is trying to make sense of something new and emotionally complex. This hybrid form sounds very strange and irrational in the terms of normative logic. Yet, out of this very 'crazy-sounding' language, Luke tends to come to very sane and personally grounded conclusions.

One image that I have had lately is that metaphact processing is a lot like deaf sign language. If you knew nothing of deaf sign language and saw a person using it on the bus, they might seem 'crazy'. But once people understand deaf sign language they find that it is a very eloquent form of communication and a thing of beauty in its own right. By listening to Luke's metaphact process, I am learning his language instead of insisting that he come over to mine. We [8] have developed this understanding of metaphact process from intensive analysis of the sessions of one client—Luke—which may seem to be slender grounds for the development of such a generalized model. But Luke's style of thinking is so characteristic of the 'thought disorder' described in the clinical psychology literature over the years that we think our understanding of Luke's process may apply to many people suffering from schizophrenia. In writing this case study, I am hoping that you will get some feeling for what this sort of metaphact process is like and see the positive potential of working with clients in this mode of experiencing.

LUKE'S BACKGROUND

When I first saw Luke, he was in his mid-thirties. Luke is a Caucasian man who grew up in a prosperous Midwestern, Irish-American family. In his late teens, during his third year at a competitive California university, Luke suffered a psychotic break. He attempted to return to the university after a period of intensive therapy and family support but soon suffered another psychotic break. For the next fifteen years he lived in a series of hospitals and supported residential settings. Therapist notes from that period suggest that sessions were engaged but often tumultuous, leading to bouts of what the therapists saw as 'counter-transference'.

At the time when I began seeing Luke, he had just moved to Chicago to live closer to his father and had entered Sheffield House, a high-quality supported residential setting in Chicago. Luke's medication had been changed to Clozaril shortly before he came to Chicago, a change that both Luke and his family thought had been helpful. A Sheffield House staff member came with him to the first therapy session. Luke seemed quiet and a little confused, but he had been in therapy before and was quite ready to participate in therapy sessions.

---

8. The development of the conceptual models has been greatly assisted by textual analyses of Luke's process conducted within the doctoral research projects of the following students of the Illinois School of Professional Psychology: Jim Collins, Kim Mandel, Sheila Senn, Chin Teoh, Judith Trytten and Robin Young. Judith Trytten conducted the first numerical research on hypotheses relating to Luke.

EARLY THERAPY

When I first met Luke, he tended to wear an incongruous mix of clothes that would make him look odd to the casual observer. His formal suit coat often had numerous 'support your local police' buttons on it and he often wore a number of colorful braided bracelets on his wrists. Sometimes he would complete the outfit with a baseball cap turned around backwards.

I began therapy trying to understand Luke and to express my understanding to him. Often Luke would start sessions with fairly long descriptions of concrete events, such as what restaurant he had gone to for lunch and exactly what he ate. But soon he would enter into descriptions of situations and reactions in very individual language. In the early days he described his problem as being 'the pain of the open road'. He felt quite normal to himself and was confused and hurt when people used the word 'schizophrenic' or 'mentally ill' to describe him. Instead, he thought that maybe, since he had gone to college for a while in the South, he was a 'southern gentleman'. And he suspected that people in the North just had trouble understanding southern gentlemen.

Sometime in these early sessions I realized that, when I paraphrased what Luke said, he wasn't clear about what I meant. For example, if he said that he was 'angry' and I responded that he was 'mad', he would say something like 'I don't know doctor, you know more about these things than I do'. So I moved more and more to following Prouty's advice in relation to contact reflections— trying to stay as close to Luke's actual words as I could—while still trying to really feel them inside of myself. Here's a small interchange:

Client: ... Yeah, ah, mentally I'm just trying to get rid of the course.

Therapist: Sure.

C: Which is where I am in the scheme of things, basically.

T: Um hum. Just trying to get rid of the course, mentally.

C: Uh huh.

T: Out of your mind?

C: Yep, out of the back, whatever.

T: Uh hum. Out of the back, whatever it is.

Early in my work with Luke, I would often understand the words Luke was using without understanding exactly what the words meant to him. What was the 'course' and why would he want to get rid of it? Yet, in this segment, you can see that when I changed his words from 'mentally' to 'out of your mind' Luke seems to get confused and needs to clarify that he means out of the 'back of his mind'. In the early days, if I asked questions for clarification, things tended to get even more confused. Luke would tend to freeze and say that he didn't want to 'talk about that'.

Yet I found that when I just stayed with his words things would start to become clearer to me. For example, it turned out that the 'course' was something bad that happened

145

in California, right before the psychotic break that related to the 'boodeyism'. Luke had been on a retreat in transcendental meditation that took him into some altered states that seemed to slide into more and more strange experiences and led to his being taken away in an ambulance. I realized after a while that, in Luke's usage, the word 'course' referred to the whole set of California experiences that had been new and tempting but that he felt were inconsistent with his Catholic upbringing. And, since these pleasurable and tempting California experiences led to the total trauma and confusion of a psychotic break, Luke understandably thought that they were something to stay away from.

Surprisingly, at some point in Luke's therapy I realized that I understood a great deal of what he was saying. Luke uses words like 'the course' in very stable ways. Often a concrete part of a troubling situation comes to stand for the whole situation and for other situations that feel the same way.[9] So, for example, if Luke is concerned that someone's behavior is too profligate or loose, he is likely to observe that that person seems to be under the influence of 'the course'. You can maybe see that I was starting to think almost like an anthropologist who is trying to understand the ways of a person from a foreign tribe. I was not thinking, 'What subconscious meaning do these words have according to some theory of depth psychology'. And I certainly wasn't thinking, 'These are random, nonsensical results of malfunctioning brain chemistry'. Rather, I was trying to understand, 'How does Luke use words and how does his inner logic work?' And since I was staying very close to Luke's own words in my responses to him, I had a lot of time to observe how Luke put thoughts together.

I started to notice that Luke often seemed to have trouble narrowing down to normatively sensible, clearly defined units to analyze personal situations and he had trouble attaching the units he did come to with normative, sensible logic. This seemed to be particularly true when Luke was struggling to make sense of situations that were emotionally loaded, but not-yet-clear. Yet, I found that these same statements often were eloquently expressive if I translated them into metaphors in my own mind. I began to think that when Luke is actively processing experience he really doesn't sense a difference, as a normatively functioning person would, between clearly defined units and metaphors.[10]

Let me give an example. One day, Luke made the following observations (slightly condensed here):

> The trouble with the world is that there are too many Spaniards. My father is a Spaniard. When he talks, I only understand about a third of what he says. I think that that's because he comes from another country. On the other hand, you seem to understand me perfectly well. That must be because we come from the same country.

---

9. J Collins (2003) has called this process of using a part of the situation to describe the whole situation as well as other situations that bear some similarity 'metasynecdoche'.

10. A number of writers such as Gregory Bateson (1972) and Michael Eigen (1986) have noticed this confusion of fact and metaphor in schizophrenic thought disorders but they have tended not to see the positive processing potential of this sort of experience.

This *sounds* as if Luke was speaking about clearly defined units (or facts) and clearly defined causal relations. Luke observes that his father *is* a Spaniard and that his trouble understanding his father comes about *because* his father is from another country. Luke seems to be working hard to make some kind of cause–effect sense out of the phenomena at hand.

Yet, notably, Luke's whole train of thought (that seems so unreasonable when seen as a rendition of facts and causes) would make sense if it were reformulated in terms of the kinds of broad similarities characteristic of metaphors or similes rather than facts and causes. Thus, a person might quite sensibly say: 'The trouble in the world is that too many people *behave as if they were* Spaniards. I feel *as if* my father is like that. He *seems as if* he comes from another country. He *might as well* be speaking Spanish; I only understand about a third of what he says. Somehow, you and I *seem like* we come from the same country. You seem to understand me perfectly well'.

Metaphacts really are a hybrid of more ordinary facts and more ordinary metaphors. Luke doesn't seem to have the metaphoric distance that would let him clearly understand that a word or image is 'like' the situation at hand, yet he doesn't expect metaphacts to have the kind of inalterability that would be typical of facts. This metaphact logic seems to get in the way of ordinary cause and effect thinking much more than they interfere with metaphoric thinking, since metaphors are about broad similarities and don't require sharp definition. When Luke holds a metaphact image in mind it tends to draw other related scenes, images and feelings to his mind; whether or not Luke has the metaphoric distance to clarify to himself, whether it is a figure of speech or a literal fact.

This new understanding of metaphacts deepened my sense of empathic connection with Luke a great deal. Now, very often, I could feel beyond the surface of Luke's words. I was not just hearing that Luke thinks his father comes from Spain (in spite of the fact that he is really an American). I started to understand that when Luke states things in metaphacts that *he* doesn't hold them quite as literal facts, but he doesn't think of them as metaphors either. He is communicating in a whole different language. With this understanding of metaphacts, I could feel with Luke as to what it must be like to sense that your parent is totally foreign to you and impossible to understand. Things that had seemed like random shifts of topic suddenly were sensible extensions of themes that Luke was exploring. I started getting the point of stories and finding the same jokes to be funny. I remember thinking that if people saw us happily talking away, they might have trouble knowing which one of us was schizophrenic!

A second shift in my empathy for Luke came from my beginning to grasp what it is like to try to make sense of life if you really can't use factual logic to work with personally significant, emotionally unclear issues. So, what would it be like to think about an issue like 'death', if you really had being 'literally dead', in the same category as various death-like experiences, such as being 'dead on your feet'? Here's another short segment from a time when Luke's father was hospitalized and a few weeks away from his ultimate death. Luke's brother had implied that their father might not make it and Luke was quite offended.

> C: *Huh uh, exactly. Huh, plus I don't think Dad is going to die for many years, and he may even outlive me, if you will, (Sure) in terms of the spirituality. (Um hum) But, uh, the church seems to believe that if you keep receiving Holy Communion, and maybe*

saying an occasional prayer, that, you know, one can actually live forever, in a way. (Um hum) My mother, as you know.

T: *Believed that. (Yeah, and …) and the church seems to believe that if you take Holy Communion, and some things like that, you may really live forever. (Yeah) And you've got to think with your Dad, that he may live for a very long time, he may outlive you. (Yeah) So in some ways it sounds like William was implying that he might not live very long.*

C: *Yeah. So these things were very upsetting for me, you know (Yes) um.*

T: *Um, you don't like to hear him say things like that.*

Using metaphact logics, Luke is quite unsure what does happen when people die. He notes that people get put into boxes underground and says that he thinks that he wouldn't like that to happen to him. But in a metaphact way, people seem to be gone, but not gone, since they still talk to him as voices and communicate to him through pictures. Luke commented at one point that he hoped that his father got out of the coffin once in a while and took trips to Las Vegas.

In all of this I started to feel into how unsafe the world would be if you couldn't distinguish facts from metaphors in a clear way. For example, what it would be like if you felt a little upset but definitely not 'crazy' and people came to drag you away in an ambulance? What would it feel like if a person in the coffee shop smiled at you and you couldn't use logic to make sense of what that meant, and you never knew when any change might mean that the ambulance would come again?

I began to sense a typical rhythm in Luke's sessions. Luke often begins by chatting a bit, but fairly quickly gets to a subject that is bothering him, much in the way that a higher functioning client might. As he explores the subject more deeply, he often comes to a flurry of metaphact language. His worst fears often have to do with the concern that if *anything* goes wrong in his life this may be the start of another psychotic crisis, with ambulances and hospitals following shortly. This pondering of his worst fears often leads to a series of scenes, images, memories and the like that hone in more exactly on what bothers Luke about the specific situation at hand. For example, a situation in which a girl smiled at him on the train led Luke to a series of memories of times in which people had smiled at him when their real intentions weren't friendly. One of these was the paramedic who smiled at him before he tackled him and took him off in the ambulance. Another was of times in college when girls seemed friendly, but reacted badly when Luke tried to approach them. Notably, these scenes are linked by their broad felt similarity rather than by cause and effect logic. Still, this progression of metaphoric similarities allows Luke to become clear about what is really worrying him about the initial situation.

Sometimes just naming his reactions seems to resolve them. At other times, after pondering scenes like these he comes up with a sense of the crux of things. These 'crux' statements tend to be personally grounded, sensible and expressed in normative language. For example, after pondering a lunch with his father in intense metaphact language,

Luke became clear that he was bothered by his father's disapproval of his smoking. Then he said, in very normative English, that smoking was his only vice and he was really unwilling to stop. He thought that his father drank too much and that they each should be entitled to one vice. In addition, he thought that his father seemed unhappy, and maybe *he* needed to be in therapy.

THE THERAPEUTIC RELATIONSHIP

I felt comfortable with being in a therapeutic relationship with Luke from the very beginning. I sensed fairly quickly that something good happened when I stayed close to Luke's exact words, even though it was quite puzzling to me how the process worked. (And, contrary to my worst fears, Luke never seemed likely to explode or to lose control during sessions.) The words I had for myself in the early sessions were 'crazy thoughts that seem to lead to sane conclusions'. My main difficulty was keeping my concentration on Luke's exact words when I didn't know what the words meant to him. Often I would take a break in the middle of a session to get another cup of coffee, just so that I could have a minute to stretch my legs and clear my head.

Some weeks into our therapy relationship, though, I realized that Luke found the process confusing since it was so different from his previous therapies. He commented that in his previous therapies he had a 'boss' and I didn't seem to be behaving like a boss. He wondered what was going on and what he was supposed to be doing. I was aware by this time that the factual explanations that others offered Luke often left him very confused. I wanted to respond authentically but in his terms. So I commented that what people usually did in this kind of therapy was to talk about their thoughts and their feelings, and that this kind of talking about your thoughts and feelings often helped with the 'pain of the open road'. This explanation seemed to relieve his mind and left him free to proceed.

I also realized in the first several months that when Luke was afraid that he had offended me (for example, if he cancelled a session) he tended to have frightening hallucinations. (I would now interpret these hallucinations as metaphacts. When he thought I was angry he felt 'as if' devils were attacking him.) So I made it a practice to call him if he didn't make it to a session to have a friendly chat in which I could agree with his reasons for not coming. Over time, Luke became very attached to our session times and now very rarely cancels. At one point Luke's father suggested that he should cut back on the therapy sessions to have more time available for vocational rehabilitation. Luke told him in no uncertain terms that we were doing important work and that his father was not to interfere.

Still, Luke remained quite uncertain as to just why the sessions helped. Once he said that he wasn't sure what we were doing, but that his thoughts seemed to be clearer at the end of sessions. At another time he commented that what we were doing must be working because the police were behaving better. Luke began to use the Counseling Center and our therapy relationship as a self-soothing image. For example, when I was away on a trip, he commented that he was doing OK because he realized that he could just send his spirit to the Center and feel OK. He was also reassured that my spirit had been doing handsprings on the lawn around Sheffield House.

My own interpretation of this was that we had succeeded in creating a space of safety between us. Luke could feel confident that whatever he was feeling or thinking was going to be OK at the Center. And, if things seemed confusing and alarming, they tended to get clearer in our sessions and to feel better at the end. At the same time there was very little pressure in our relationship. In this one relationship, he could speak in his own metaphact language and expect to be understood. And he didn't have the confusion of trying to make sense of another person's non-metaphact language.

On my side, the more I became attuned to metaphact language, the more I came to enjoy Luke's way of expressing himself and to be moved by his personal struggles. The images that Luke uses are richly poetic. In any given session I am likely to be touched by the way that various scenes and images come together in a new understanding for Luke. I don't make this sense of pleasure happen in any intentional way. But I imagine that Luke feels it. I suspect that it helps him that I hear what he is thinking and feeling, as it is expressed in his own internal language, and that I both understand and appreciate him in that language.

LONG-TERM CHANGES IN LUKE'S STYLE OF PROCESSING

In my observation of Luke, he seems to have made a great deal of progress in finding ways to process effectively using metaphact language. His process is slower than a more normative client's process might be since he needs to make sense of many aspects of situations that would be processed quasi-automatically by most people. (For example, a server in the coffee shop who smiles at him can be quite puzzling to him.) And, given the difficulty forming clear units and causes in metaphact language, Luke sometimes has trouble making sense of particular logical aspects of personal situations. (For example he has difficulty understanding why people would think that smoking cigarettes would give a person cancer.) But, in spite of these limitations, metaphact process is *very* effective in clarifying Luke's understanding of what is bothering him, why it bothers him and what he would like to have happen. You might compare this to the situation of a person who has lost a great deal of his or her vision who finds alternative ways to orient themselves—perhaps by intensifying attention to touch, or hearing, or by reading in Braille.

I also have the sense that Luke is slowly restoring more normative processing capacities in some significant ways. Luke has greatly increased his ability to understand another person's point of view while keeping that person's personality and situation separate from his own personality and reactions to the situation. He has gradually come to have a more normative understanding of some large and emotionally loaded concepts such as 'schizophrenia'. And he has started to notice when other people are doing things that would seem 'odd' in social situations.

He has become very adept at using unit logics in relation to a number of phenomena that used to fall into the logical confusion of metaphacts. For example, Luke now takes great pleasure in figuring out what the weather is in different states and how weather patterns might be moving geographically. Earlier he would have tended to blend thoughts about the weather with cultural characteristics or his emotional responses to different parts of the country. (For example, in earlier years, he might have thought that it was hot in Moscow because the Russians were 'red'.) In recent years I have found that I can say the point of a story in my own words without confusing Luke, and that he is very able to answer questions about what he means or how he came to a particular conclusion. So, to continue the earlier metaphor, it is as if Luke had regained his sight enough to see the broad outlines of things around him, while still needing to use Braille or a cane to orient himself more exactly.

METAPHACT PROCESS AND THE BRAIN: SOME SPECULATIONS[11]

A number of theorists have noted that in 'normal' processing people pull together a number of quite different, even contradictory, styles of thinking. While both the right and left hemispheres of the brain are involved to some degree in virtually all thinking, the hemispheres have strengths in quite different modes of thought. Rotenberg (1994) notes:

> The basic function of the left hemisphere is a consecutive analysis of information, whether verbal or nonverbal while the function of the right hemisphere is a single state processing of many elements of information as a unitary whole. This makes possible rapid single state grasping of the essence of an object or phenomenon even before it is analyzed.

The frontal lobes of the brain have an executive function, drawing on different kinds of brain functioning as needed in different situations.[12] Notably, research has found that tasks that are new and unclear to research subjects bring more frontal lobe activity and also tend to engage the right hemisphere more strongly than the left hemisphere. More practised tasks go more strongly to the left hemisphere and have less intense frontal lobe involvement.

Some theorists have suggested that voices and hallucinations are aspects of right hemispheric functioning that are ordinarily inhibited by the left hemisphere.[13] Julian Jaynes (1976) suggests that hearing voices and seeing hallucinations may have been characteristic of early humans, only to have disappeared from everyday experience as the more verbal, logical left hemisphere increased in size and dominance. In any case,

---

11. For a more in-depth analysis of metaphact process, thought disorder and the brain, see Warner (2007).
12. See E. Goldberg (2001) pp. 69–85 for an analysis of the integrating activity of the frontal lobes in relation to the right and left hemispheres of the brain.
13. See L. Cozolino (2004) pp. 119–21 for a summary of this view of the role of the right hemisphere in relation to hallucinations and voices.

voices and hallucinations seem to us to have the same metaphact quality that verbal images do.

Ordinary thinking—especially thinking about feelings, intentions, personal qualities and the like—involves an exquisite mix of these two modes of thought. For example, a woman might think: 'This person I'm dating has all of the qualities I've always thought I wanted. He is solid, considerate, and very, very attentive. But somehow I feel as if I'm suffocating whenever I'm with him. I just don't understand why I would feel that way…' In a left hemisphere style, the qualities that this woman is looking for fit into clearly defined categories—'solid', 'considerate', 'attentive'. She could probably talk about what he is doing that fits the ordinary definition of those categories. At the same time, in a more right hemisphere mode of process, she has an overall feel of the relationship, captured by the metaphor 'suffocating'. Without any special effort she knows the difference between these two modes of thought. She knows that she means 'considerate' as a label for a culturally defined phenomenon and that 'suffocating' is a metaphor. Feeling 'as if' she is suffocating, is very different from 'really' suffocating.

So, what is going on with Luke? He seems to be trying to process novel experiences in his life in the way any ordinary person would, by touching into experiences that are felt but not yet clear. Eugene Gendlin[14] calls these sorts of experiences the person's 'felt sense' of a situation. Yet, at these times of Luke's most active processing, something unusual seems to occur. Luke seems to be trying to apply the sort of clear logic that is appropriate to left brain processing to the more global wholes that typically emerge from right brain process, without having any sense of metaphoric distance as he does this. In the process, the two styles of thinking come together in a complex hybrid, having some of the qualities of more ordinary factual thinking and some of the qualities of more global, metaphoric or felt-sense thinking.

If, as I suspect, this sort of metaphact process happens at the level of the brain it wouldn't do much good to just tell someone to stop thinking this way. The main way that a person could stop metaphact process would be to stop paying attention to anything unclear or emotionally complex. But, in the process of not thinking about aspects of their experience that are not-yet-clear, the person would be left without any way to come to a personally integrated, authentic version of what they are feeling, wanting or intending. If I am correct—that metaphact process is the primary avenue that a schizophrenic person has available with which to clarify personal reactions—usual therapeutic strategy or ignoring or discouraging 'schizophrenic-sounding' talk is exceedingly misguided.

---

14. Gendlin has developed a very sophisticated philosophical and psychological understanding of human experiencing as it is 'carried forward' in the creation of meaning. See, for example, Gendlin (1964, 1968 and 1995). Recent work can be found on the website www.focusing.org.

QUESTIONS RAISED BY THIS STYLE OF THERAPY

I have found that when I describe this style of therapy, practitioners schooled in other theories often have questions. Let me respond to some of the most frequent ones in case they might be coming up for you.

1. ISN'T LUKE JUST USING METAPHACT PROCESS AS A WAY OF RUNNING AWAY FROM REALITY?

It is striking to me that Luke doesn't use metaphacts when he is avoiding subjects. Luke moves into metaphact process when he has turned his attention to aspects of his experience that are not yet clear and often emotionally loaded. His engaging with metaphact process leads him to positive processing steps: exploring his fears; differentiating reactions that had been previously unarticulated; designing positive strategies to handle situations and the like.

The assumption that psychotic experience *results from* the person's fears of facing reality is a very old one with roots in early psychoanalytic theory. Now that we know more about the biological changes often involved in various forms of schizophrenia we should at least question this assumption. Yet, even humanistically-oriented therapists often state that psychosis *always* comes from an inability to face existential challenges as if this were an established fact.

I am more inclined to think of Luke as a person who has courageously struggled to create a satisfying life in the face of a substantial disability (the severe difficulty in distinguishing facts and metaphors when dealing with new material). And I am reinforced in my belief that the human inclination to make sense is so strong that the mind will struggle to find alternative routes if the more normative ways of making sense are blocked.

2. AREN'T YOU AFRAID THAT YOU ARE JUST REINFORCING A PSYCHOTIC, THOUGHT-DISORDERED WAY OF THINKING?

I am struck by the fact that the 'crux' statements that Luke comes up with in the middle of metaphact processing are not only personally grounded and realistic, they *tend to be expressed in normative language.* Also, observers have noted that when Luke is in public, he tends not to speak in schizophrenic language. (Luke once referred to this as 'keeping his cards close to his chest'.) Luke seems to need the metaphact language when he is trying to make sense of things that are felt but that are not yet clear. But once he has clarified thoughts, feelings, wishes, intentions and the like, he seems to be able to bring them into more normative conversations in ordinary language. The fact that Luke has so strikingly increased the number and quality of his social interactions over the years suggests that his use of metaphact language in therapy helps rather than hinders his ability to conduct everyday relationships using more normative language.

3. COULDN'T YOU JUST EXPLAIN TO LUKE THAT HE IS BLURRING FACTS AND METAPHORS AND TEACH HIM TO THINK IN MORE NORMATIVE WAYS?

I've never tried this, but I don't think that it would work. I've heard Luke describe innumerable interactions in which Sheffield House staff or family members try to explain emotionally loaded subjects (like why he shouldn't smoke) with normative cause-effect logics. Luke feels quite confused by these explanations. He takes in the explanations through the same metaphact lens with which he takes in other novel information, blurring facts and metaphors. Often, rather than making things clear to him, these explanations lead him to give up on understanding what is going on. Instead, he just tries to fake it, trying to meet other people's expectations. Or he stubbornly refuses to go along while not being willing to explain why.

4. SHOULDN'T YOU BE TEACHING LUKE SOCIAL SKILLS AND TRYING TO GET HIM TO BE MORE SOCIALLY ENGAGED THAN HE IS?

Pushing for social activity and training in social skill may work for some clients, but it doesn't seem to have helped Luke. I have spent innumerable sessions hearing Luke's reactions to situations in which staff members tried to bring about sociable activities. Sheffield House has sometimes had programs in which residents were obliged to select a fixed number of social activities in which to participate. Luke has almost always hated these activities.

In one session, Luke spent a lot of time puzzling over an event called 'coffee house' in which Sheffield House residents were expected to sit and listen to music together and dance. Luke commented that the whole event was puzzling. He hated the event, other residents hated the event, and the staff seemed to hate it too. So Luke came to the conclusion that there must be some forces in the sky pulling their strings to make them all do it. These forced social activities seem to just get Luke to go through the motions of sociable activity without having any feelings of sociability.

On the other hand, I am struck by the way that genuine and spontaneously sociable feelings emerge when Luke is able to process his feelings about life situations in his own language. My ideal residential or day program would have a stable and friendly environment with good food and with staff who know clients well. In addition, it would offer person-centered therapy and a variety of activities to any participants who wanted them. But it would not require residents to participate in activities if they didn't personally want to.

5. YOUR THERAPY WITH LUKE HAS GONE ON FOR A VERY LONG TIME. IS THIS A REALISTIC MODE OF THERAPY IN AN ERA OF MANAGED CARE?

I think that the debilitating effects of schizophrenia are often more drastic than those of having a heart attack or stroke, given the excruciating experiences, social isolation, homelessness and suicide that often come with schizophrenia. Yet, in industrialized countries, we spend hundreds of thousands of dollars on physical ailments without batting an eyelid. Judging from my experience with Luke, I think that for many clients, ongoing therapy that supports metaphact processing could make the difference between a tormented, isolated life and a life that, even if somewhat restricted, is genuinely engaged and satisfying.

REFERENCES

Bateson, G (1972) *Steps to an Ecology of Mind.* Northvale, NJ: Jason Aronson Inc.

Brune, M (2005) 'Theory of Mind' in schizophrenia: A review of the literature. *Schizophrenia Bulletin, 31,* 121–42.

Collins, J (2003) Narrative Theory and Schizophrenia: The construction of self via non-normative processing. Unpublished Clinical Research Project. Illinois School of Professional Psychology of Argosy University/Chicago.

Cozolino, L (2004) *The Neuroscience of Psychotherapy: Building and rebuilding the human brain.* New York: WW Norton.

Eigen, M (1986) *The Psychotic Core.* Northvale, NJ: Jason Aronson Inc.

Gendlin, ET (1964) A theory of personality change. In P Worchel and D Byrne (eds) *Personality Change* (pp. 100–48). New York: John Wiley and Sons.

Gendlin, ET (1968) The experiential response. In E Hammer (ed) *The Use of Interpretation in Treatment* (pp. 208–27). New York: Grune and Stratton.

Gendlin, ET (1995) Crossing and dipping: Some terms for approaching the interface between natural understanding and logical formulation. *Minds and Machines, 5,* 547–60.

Goldberg, E (2001) *The Executive Brain.* Oxford: Oxford University Press.

Jaynes, J (1976) *The Origin of Consciousness in the Breakdown of the Bicameral Mind.* Boston: Houghton Mifflin.

Karon, BP and VandenBos, GR (1981) *Psychotherapy of Schizophrenia: The treatment of choice.* Northvale, NJ: Jason Aronson Inc.

Prouty, G (1994) *Theoretical Evolutions in Person-Centered/Experiential Psychotherapy: Applications to schizophrenic and retarded psychoses.* Westport, CT: Praeger.

Prouty, G, Van Werde, D and Pörtner, M (2002) *Pre-Therapy: Reaching contact-impaired clients.* Ross-on-Wye: PCCS Books.

Rogers, CR, Gendlin, ET, Kiesler, DJ and Truax, CB (1967) (eds) *The Therapeutic Relationship and its Impact: A study of psychotherapy with schizophrenics.* Madison: University of Wisconsin Press.

Rotenberg, V (1994) An integrative psychophysiological approach to brain hemisphere functions in schizophrenia. *Neuroscience and Biobehavioral Review, 18,* 487–95.

Thase, ME and Jindal, RD (2004) Combining psychotherapy and psychopharmacology for treatment of mental disorders. In AE Bergin, SL Garfield and M J Lambert (eds) *Bergin and Garfield's Handbook of Psychotherapy and Behavior Change, 5th edn.* (pp. 742–66). New York: John Wiley & Sons.

Torrey, EF (1983) *Surviving Schizophrenia: A family manual.* New York: Harper and Row.

Warner, MS (2006) Toward an integrated person-centered theory of wellness and psychopathology. *Person-Centered and Experiential Psychotherapies 5,* 4–20.

Warner, MS (in press) Metaphact process: A new way of understanding schizophrenic thought disorder. In G Prouty (ed) *The Pre-Therapy Reader.* Ross-on-Wye: PCCS Books.

CHAPTER 14

THE IMPACT OF THE NON-DIRECTIVE ATTITUDE: A DEMONSTRATION INTERVIEW WITH CARL ROGERS

BRIAN E. LEVITT

Carl Rogers left behind an enormous legacy in written articles, chapters, books, audio and video recordings of psychotherapy and demonstration sessions. He is cited as the first to publish an entire transcript of a psychotherapy session (Rogers, 1942). A transcript of a demonstration interview with Carl Rogers and Gina (a code name), which took place about forty years later on 28 September 1983 sits in a box in the Manuscript Division of the Library of Congress in the United States (Rogers, 1983).[1] Along with this transcript is a letter from Gina to Carl, and this letter makes it clear that they both intended this demonstration to be published. Gina herself transcribed the interview, and she concludes her heartfelt letter to Carl by writing, 'Thank you for helping humans to understand themselves better!' What follows in this chapter, almost twenty-five years later, is the entire transcript of that interview, as put together by Gina, along with my own explorations of what transpired in the interview in the context of non-directive theory and practice.

When reading a transcript such as this, it is tempting to pick apart Rogers' responses and to critique the apparent accuracy of his empathic understanding. However, an analysis of empathic understanding responses has the potential to reinforce the mistaken notion that non-directive therapy is a method, a particular type of responding that can be taught and learned as a technique. When trying to understand the non-directive attitude, such an analysis is often a dead end, a fool's game that can lead to gross misunderstandings of what is actually occurring between the therapist and client. There is much more contained in a therapist's responses, which are really only a byproduct of the non-directive attitude, than we can see in printed words on a page. A transcript cannot carry with it Carl's and Gina's body language as they interact. It cannot capture nuances in tone of voice or pace. Nor can it carry a full experience for the reader of Carl's presence with Gina, or Gina's presence with Carl. Carl's words do not necessarily give us, as readers, the attitudes and deep warmth that are carried in them. These are just some of the important subtleties that the reader cannot hope to ever fully grasp in the words printed on the page. Furthermore, it is clear from Rogers (1959) that the client's *perception* of the therapist's empathic understanding of, and unconditional regard for, the client are what is truly important. Ultimately, whether a response carries a high

---

1. Reprinted here with the kind permission of Natalie Rogers.

degree of empathic understanding is up to Gina, and no one else. As such, I would ask you, the reader, to put aside any efforts to analyze the accuracy of Rogers' empathic understanding responses, and focus more on how Gina appears to be receiving Carl in their interactions and how she comes to further understand herself.

DEMONSTRATION INTERVIEW ON 28 SEPTEMBER 1983

Carl: I think that we should take a moment or two, I want to get quiet within myself and you were saying that you felt uneasy about this too, and so let's just take a moment or two to get quiet within ourselves so that we can really have an interview.

Pause

I don't know what you would like to talk about, but I'm more than willing to listen.

Gina 1: Thank you. I would like to tell you something what happened to me a few weeks ago, and it was quite an experience I had in myself, and I thought meanwhile that I came over it so far. I think I learned a lot on one hand, but on the other hand I feel a bit stuck, and to explain that, I have to tell you the story that happened first. And I feel a bit foolish about it, and for me it is quite a risk to tell it. But on the other hand it is a chance to tell it and so I'll do it.

Carl 1: Even in spite of the risk you'll take a chance of telling the incident and how you felt two ways about it.

Gina 2: Yes. I see a chance in it as well. It has something to do with the political situation we are all living in now. We are all very much afraid about a third world war. And oddly enough a few weeks ago it happened by coincidence that ... an astrologist came into our house in order to see my husband because he is interested in astrology ... and he knows quite a lot about this Hindu astrology, which isn't that well-known in Germany. But it is supposed to be very precise. He came into our house and delivered some books and he said by the way, I'll get you this now, because I'm leaving next week to Australia. I asked him why and he said I'm emigrating because I'm expecting the third world war. And that really hit me.

Carl 2: Hmm. That would be terrifying.

Gina 3: It was terrifying, and at first I thought by myself, 'I don't want to listen to him.' But then I got such an urge to ask him more about it ... and so he told us all what he knows about, from the astrologist point of view and he used some prophesies as well from seers, who lived 200 years ago in Germany, and it is all written down. And he described it all so vividly ... really, it put me off totally.

Carl 3: It just seemed as though here was a lot of evidence.

Gina 4: Ja. And … after he … anyway, he told us as well he would expect that … he described it you know, he said, 'The Russians will definitely march into Germany and they will come very soon.' And he described it so far very convincing, very vividly … regarding the whole situation you know, concerning the missiles, the Pershing 2, and he said, 'The Russians will not allow the stationing in Germany.' and all that. And I came more and more to the point that I believed it, and—well, I had three hard nights after that and I couldn't sleep at all. And I got really sick somehow, it hit me so deeply, because suddenly I felt my deepest fear and I was confronted with that.

Carl 4: Hmm. The thing you'd been afraid of the most suddenly was right there and (Gina: Yes.) made you sick and you couldn't sleep (Gina: Yes.) it really just terrified you.

Gina 5: Yes. You know the war danger I ignored before, you know, I thought there is something, but … maybe it never happens. But suddenly it became so close.

Carl 5: Very real.

Gina 6: Very real, yes. And the peculiar thing was that he said it will happen very soon— he meant inside four weeks—and well, I, I was so confused about it, what to do and all that, and strangely enough at the same time as he expected this even, my husband had a business trip to London. And so I decided to go with him, and see what happens. So during the next weeks, I really went into myself, they … er … we rehearsed the catastrophe … (I can't translate the meaning.) [Gina is transcribing this herself, and cannot understand what she said in German. Ed.] *We felt that it would happen and what does that mean to us. Anyway we had to go to that time, and all went through my mind during those days it was really full of despair and fear, an … and it meant a lot you know. Everything suddenly went upside down, you know, I went …*

Carl 6: It was just a very traumatic experience where everything came together that you had feared.

Gina 7: Yes, but it was only in myself, you know, and, of course my husband was involved, but he took it differently. And …

Carl 7: For you it really got you inside.

Gina 8: Yes. And I wanted to throw up everything what I needed before, what I loved before, and I thought what a load of rubbish I'd collected, I don't need more than two cups and all that, you know. Suddenly I found out what possession means, that it means nothing in such a situation. And I was so full of fear, because I thought if it happens I have to go because I can't stand it here, I … I can't stand the cruelty, horror and wretchedness I'm facing. It wasn't the idea of being afraid to die, because everybody has to die one fine day. You know, but I felt so stuck, I … I thought … I can't die and I can't live. It was something like that.

Carl 8: You felt paralyzed, it sounds like. (Gina: Yes.) It really wasn't the fear of death; that you can accept. But here it was neither life nor death; you were just stuck in the middle.

Gina 9: Yes. And that made me not sleep for a few nights. And after that I thought OK, I felt it somehow and faced the idea of emigrating, of leaving because you aren't able to stand it.

Carl 9: You mean you sort of shut it out of mind after that?

Gina 10: No. No it changed so far that I said, 'OK, it might happen.' (Carl: I see.) But I won't face it when it happens, I'm going to escape.

Carl 10: I see. That became your belief that (Gina: Yes.) somehow you would escape when it did happen.

Gina 11: Yes. That was true to that time for me. And anyway we went to England to that time, and it was really an extraordinary trip to have this in your mind, you know, the people, the relatives in London—my husband is English—on the one hand they had a good laugh about it, you know, well, 'We finally got you to London because of the Russians,' on the other hand they took us seriously, and the night before it happened, we had a last meal together, all these things, you know, and we … it was a kind of paranoiac situation. And anyway the Russians didn't come and we came back. But …

Carl 11: It sounds as though in England it was both a joke and very serious. (Gina: Yes.) And that adds to the confusion. And then it didn't happen and you came back.

Gina 12: It didn't happen, and we came back, and somewhat I felt very embarrassed about it, you know, after that, well, stupid me believing those prophesies and all that, and why did I take it so seriously. But on the other hand I came back and felt nothing had changed. We are still living in such a threatening situation, and that is still the situation now. Afterwards, what I needed to do first, not to think about it anymore, not to speak about it anymore—and what I did, I gave a good cleaning to the whole house, and needed to redo everything, it was quite an impulse. And then later on, after that I came to another decision, well, that if it would really happen—and you know meanwhile what happened to that aeroplane the Russians shot down—if it started again like that a bit, I thought next time I won't be moved. Next time I (Carl: I won't leave.) I won't emigrate, I won't escape.

Carl 12: Next time I'll stay there.

Gina 13: I'll stay there and stand it. But still, it is something I, I'm so stuck in it. I don't know how to handle it, because I found out there are two sides of it. One hand it's the real threat from outside which you read in every newspaper, the other side is how to handle it with my person. What do I do with it? And I'm so afraid that I'm going on the ignore trip again. You know, on my ignoring trip again.

Carl 13: So there's two sides. One is the very real threat from outside, but the other question is, how am I going to deal with it within myself? You feel I don't want to just shut it out, I don't want to ignore it because that still leaves you uncertain how to count your way in the world.

Gina 14: Yes, and I think it is something deeper. I guess it must be something really existential in myself which I haven't touched yet. And I was already thinking, I mean I'm not the type who is a member of a demonstration, I think I might feel lost when a lot of people are demonstrating for peace, although I'm with them in my thoughts. I think being able to do something about it at all must be first to get to know something of this deep existential question in myself. In our church around the corner, they offer three days meditation and fasting for peace. I would like to take part and don't want it as a demonstration, you know, to be read about in the newspaper the next day that a couple of people did that. I was thinking to join it to do it for myself. It will be to find a kind of peace in myself because in this fact I am still stuck.

Carl 14: I want to make sure that I'm understanding you that, anything you might do outside, like demonstrating and so on, still doesn't get you to the deeper thing in yourself (Gina: Right!) and you really like to get to that (Gina: Yes.) and if you did demonstrate it wouldn't be for the sake of publicity, it would be for the hope of getting to that deeper aspect of you.

Gina 15: Right! Exactly that! (Pause) I ... What I want for myself, you know, to get the peace, you know, that for the case ... if really something happens that ... I would be able to ... accept is the wrong word ... something between acceptation and surrender ...

Carl 15: It sounds as though you are asking something like: 'Can I possibly be at peace with myself even if this awful thing happens.' (Gina: Yes.) Somewhere between ...

Gina 16: I would like to have the power to say, 'OK, if I can't do something about it. I have ... I have to take it.' Though I would like to have some hope in me ... and some power still, just in this time ... because I think I need it and ... I need get it out too. I ...

Carl 16: And it isn't quite acceptance, and it isn't quite surrender, but you would hope to find a place within yourself that you can live with, it seems like.

Gina 17: Yes, yes! (Pause) What do we do, when this happens?

Carl 17: What did you say?

Gina 18: What do we do, when this happens? I think it is a question nobody can answer.

Carl 18: That's the question that just seems unanswerable: 'What do I do when it happens?' (Gina: Yes!) 'How do I deal with that within myself?'

Gina 19: Yes! (Pause) You know, I thought I was over it. I thought, I was a step further through this experience. But I'm so afraid, if those things happen, it all goes over and over again in me. I was so afraid and when I think about it I get again such a fear …

Carl 19: This thinking about it stirs you up and stirs you up inside with that same fear. (Gina: Yes.)

Gina 20: And I have got no answer yet, and I don't think that I'll ever find one. What I just found out through talking with friends about it, that they feel the same … But you know, you just put a lot of energy in only talking to each other about your fears. And that's it. That's all.

Carl 20: To know, that you are not alone in that fear, the others have the same kind of fear. (Gina: Yes.) (Pause)

Gina 21: At least you can name it as a fear of dying in such a way …

Carl 21: I missed the way you say that—it's a fear of dying in such a way, is that it? (Gina: Yes!) (Pause)

Gina 22: I mean, I can only take this very personal way, because I think at least it has something to do with the person who is facing this situation. And look at the people who are with me now and have to face it … And to have a hold of the fear, maybe you have to change something in yourself. That's my kind of idea of it.

Carl 22: You find yourself wishing, that you could get rid of the fear within yourself, and face it in some new way. (Gina: Yes!) (Pause) As you just sighed and let down a step a little? (Pause)

Gina 23: I get somewhat empty by talking about it.

Carl 23: Empty—and it looks as though you feel relaxed too. (Pause)

Gina 24: I feel relaxed for the moment, because I feel that I can only come so far, you know, just facing it—it is there and I have to live with it. I'm thinking, 'OK, it is like that …'

Carl 24: You just feel, it is a reality that you live with.

Gina 25: Yes. It is reality. And I want for me to … (Pause) To get more mature about it …

Carl 25: More mature, and …

Gina 26: More wisdom. Just to live with it.

Carl 26: You want to be wise enough and mature enough to somehow live even with that. (Gina: Yes!) (Pause)

Gina 27: Yes, that's it!

Carl 27: Do you like to stop? I think we just have a few more minutes!

Gina 28: I think I would like to have a few more minutes too. I got another thought. (Pause) I would like you to let me know what you think about it. I mean the whole subject.

End of Session

Carl 28: I feel privileged to have been able to go with you so deeply into a terrible, terrible fear, and I admire the fact that you have come out with the feeling: 'I need maturity to live with that fear within myself.' I really feel very touched by that, very moved by that … (Pause) Perhaps when you feel ready, you might be willing to tell the group how this experience seemed to you, and I'll say, how it seemed to me, and then we can see, if they have questions or comments they want to make, if you are willing to hear them. (Gina: Yes.) (Pause)

Gina 29: For me you said very little to it and I was grateful for that, because it gave me the chance to look as far as I could what really happened to me. So I got contact again to that helpless feeling and confusion and ruthlessness … I found out through that, that one can't change an existential feeling like that, because it is there. And for me this is a step to know it clearly, because then I can handle with it. And I got myself sure again, I won't escape once more, I think. If it ever happens, I have to face it, I … yes, that's it.

Carl 29: Thank you very much. I felt, as I say, very deeply moved because I feel that you're speaking not only for yourself but for millions of other people too. And one thing struck me part of the way through the interview was: It is as though I was talking with a terminally ill patient, where—'cos you didn't express any hope that the situation might be changed—it was, how could you deal with it within yourself. That to me seems both marvelous and courageous—and it also fills me with enormous anger, that we can't change the external situation. It seems so stupid that in a world of intelligent people we can't change the situation. So to me it was a very moving experience, I feel very grateful to you for it. I don't particularly feel like commenting on the technical aspects of the interview, because the experience itself was so deep and potent. Thank you—and are you willing now for others to comment and question? (Gina: Yes.) If you like to raise questions or make comments, you may ...

Question from a member of the group: Gina, I didn't have the feeling that you feel better now. But I was very moved and touched too, because I have the same fears, not as horrible as yours. But my question also to Mr. Rogers is: If Gina finds peace within herself and is able to face this horrible situation we are confronted with—does this lead to passivity, especially to political passivity—or where can I find the empowerment to fight, because you said, Mr. Rogers, we cannot change the situation and I do not want to believe that! We are able to change the reality. This is a political question, I think!

Carl 30: You misunderstood me on one point: I didn't say it couldn't be changed. I said I was impressed by the fact she accepted the fact that it couldn't be changed—Personally I just finished a paper and in my talk tomorrow night I'll be trying to say some of the things that I hope might change the situation—But I really disagree very much that what Gina was showing was passivity, I don't agree with that—I think that when one is in peace within oneself it is more possible to take effective social action—And I like very much the fact that if she takes part in a demonstration it won't be just to see her name in a paper, it'll be because it feeds something in herself.

Gina 30: Right! Thank you for understanding just the right thing because I got this in my mind (at the end of the interview!) but I didn't tell it the moment I felt it. I felt: When I find that peace I get more power to do anything (in a direction I'm convinced of) whatever it is, but anything! But I didn't say it ...

Carl 31: I suspect that one reason that there are not lots of questions is that all of us feel deeply moved by the experience and that doesn't lead to quick questions. One thought that occurs to me is, that we might sit quietly for a few moments and then take a break for dinner.

DISCUSSION

A WAY OF BEING

The two essential components of Rogers' theory are the non-directive attitude and the actualizing tendency.[2] Non-directivity is an attitude held by the therapist with regard to

---

2. The non-directive attitude is given full expression in Rogers' unfolding of the therapist conditions of empathic understanding, unconditional positive regard, and congruence within the overall conditions that are necessary and sufficient for therapeutic change; see Levitt (2005).

the client's right as a separate person to have a free rein over her own process in therapy, including not only the contents and goals, but also the pace. It is a belief in her right to define herself at all times. This therapist attitude is an essential and integral part of empathic understanding, unconditional positive regard, and congruence. When discussing the concept of non-directivity, it can be hard to convince people that Carl Rogers had no method. At least, he had no method in the traditional sense of the word; no set of techniques that can be taught to others. Rather, he operated from a set of core beliefs about the value of the individual and the omnipresence of human potential. These beliefs informed him regarding how he should *be* in relation to others in order to receive and appreciate them as unique and valuable individuals. The way in which the non-directive therapist is present with the client is emphasized to the exclusion of any set of pre-ordained techniques to be used. Rogers described this way of being vis-à-vis the core conditions, which his research showed to be necessary and sufficient for therapeutic growth. He demonstrated that this way of being frees others to self-actualize; to be more fully themselves.

The actualizing tendency is a theoretical construct,[3] suggesting that all living things have a forward-moving potential for growth and positive change. The individual is 'always motivated, is always "up to something", always seeking' (Rogers, 1963: 6). This tendency towards actualizing is always being expressed, no matter how pathological a client's verbalizations, behaviors or attitudes may seem. In other words, the non-directive therapist trusts that all clients have the capacity and tendency to actualize and that this capacity is always present. The non-directive therapist expresses this basic trust in the client by following the client's direction fully and without judgment.

THE CLIENT DIRECTS THERAPY

What we see in the demonstration interview is representative of what we see across all of Rogers' therapy and demonstration sessions that were recorded. The direction for what happens and how it unfolds is in the client's hands—this is an essential feature of non-directive therapy. At the beginning of the demonstration, Carl tells Gina, 'I don't know what you would like to talk about, but I'm more than willing to listen.' We see from Carl, that any account of Gina's presenting issues is best left to her—and she unfolds this beautifully across the course of the interview and subsequent discussion. Nowhere does Rogers interfere with this unfolding, nowhere does he impose his direction on hers. In Gina 29, we see Gina reflecting on her awareness that Carl did not interfere with her process. She felt she had the space, the freedom, to explore spontaneously where she wanted and needed to go. Every step of the way, Carl is following Gina's meanings and not creating new ones or new directions. He is trying always to empathically understand Gina from her own frame while Gina directs the interview.

The client's perception of being empathically understood is paramount, along with her feeling that she is being received with unconditional positive regard. Even where it

_____

3. See Rogers (1963), Bozarth and Brodley (1991) and Brodley (1999).

might seem to us that Carl is not understanding Gina fully, it is important to recognize that she perceives him to be understanding her. At almost every turn, she spontaneously tells Rogers that he has understood her meaning by saying such things as 'yes' or 'that's it' (for instance, Gina 15, Gina 17, Gina 19, Gina 27). When his expression of meaning is very close to hers, she also seems to echo his words as she continues, as if they are on the same page in terms of the meaning for her (for example, Carl 2/Gina 3, Carl 5/Gina 6). Carl never parrots Gina. He also does not get ahead of her, though on first blush it may appear as if he does at times (Carl 2). However, if we take into consideration what Rogers has said about his approach to therapy, and we listen to what Gina tells us of her experience throughout the demonstration and in the discussion that follows it, a more complete way of seeing his responses emerges. Carl seems to be taking in, and experiencing, more than just Gina's verbal expressions as we see them on the printed page. In fact, at Carl 23 we see Carl not only being empathic to Gina's spoken language, but also to her body language. It seems that Carl is taking in the entirety of her expression, her full moment-to-moment presence throughout the interview. This deep empathic awareness appears to be informing Carl's understanding of what Gina experiences and expresses.

What is most affirming in these simple twenty-eight pairs of exchanges, with regard to the ever present human potential for growth, is the spontaneous elaboration we see in Gina's exploration. Rogers never gets ahead of her, yet she is always moving forward, always unfolding something. We can see, in her being understood and accepted for her direction and pace, a natural growth is occurring. By the end of the interview, Gina comes to a new and powerful understanding of herself. She directs the interview and her own experience.

THE THERAPIST'S MAIN GOAL—TO UNDERSTAND THE CLIENT'S MEANINGS

If the client is directing therapy, then what is the therapist doing? Generally, the non-directive therapist is always striving to be open to the client's unique direction and way of being. This requires a stance of unconditional positive regard to whatever the client brings. The therapist tries to understand the client as fully as possible as a separate individual. In order to understand a client from her own frame, the therapist must maintain the discipline to not impose his own frame or values. The therapist must see the client as a person of worth in her own right, without trying to change her. Rogers (1957) called this understanding from a non-directive stance 'empathic understanding'. Empathic understanding is an attitude, not a technique. It is embodied along with the therapist attitudes of unconditional positive regard and congruence. Rogers made it clear that there is simply no room for anything else in his mind when he tries to understand a client's frame in this non-directive way.[4] This attempt at understanding the other from her frame, and not from the therapist's frame, is essentially what the therapist is always doing.

---

4. See Rogers (1951) and Raskin (1947/2005).

What is a good empathic understanding response? Perhaps the better question is: Who decides what is a good empathic understanding response? From the perspective of the non-directive approach, the answer is obvious. The client decides. If the client feels understood, and is not jarred or set off course, then the therapist's response was a good empathic understanding response. We can see, looking at Gina's progress over 28 interactions, evidence that she feels Carl's empathic understanding responses are good— and she says so during the discussion that follows their demonstration. We might, in retrospect, pick apart Carl's empathic understanding responses, showing where they might be lacking, but this really misses the point. The point is that Gina feels understood. Something is happening in this demonstration that Gina experiences as growthful. Carl is accurate enough, and his non-directive intent is clear. This is something that Gina apparently feels in their interactions. What we are seeing is evidence of the presence of something beyond the transcript—a warm, accepting presence and sense of being understood that Gina must be experiencing beyond what we can immediately see in Carl's words in these pages.

In her letter, Gina thanks Carl for helping humans to understand themselves better. By Rogers' own accounts, this is not what he sets out to do in therapy, though he recognizes it as a consistent occurrence that follows from his way of being with others. In the demonstration, Carl is only trying to understand what Gina is experiencing and expressing as well as he can. He often expresses his understanding tentatively. In doing this, he demonstrates in a very real way his willingness to make room for her own personal power. You can almost hear Rogers saying every step along the way 'I want to make sure that I'm understanding you.' And he actually does verbalize this at Carl 14.

CARL AND GINA—THE IMPACT OF THE CLIENT ON THE NON-DIRECTIVE THERAPIST

Carl's relationship with Gina, as we have seen, is marked by his non-directive attitude, his trust in Gina's direction. This comes across in his statements, which indicate a solid empathic following. He never takes the lead, and his intent seems to be that he is trying to understand what Gina is experiencing and expressing from her perspective, not from his own. Sometimes he checks with her to make sure he has understood her meaning. As already noted, he often sounds tentative, appearing aware that he does not hold the truth for Gina. She alone holds the power to define herself.

This transcript lets us in on Carl's reactions to Gina, as we have a recording that captures their reactions after the interview. Carl expresses that he feels 'privileged' to have had the opportunity to be with Gina and follow her very personal exploration. He comes away from the encounter 'very touched ... very moved' by the way in which she comes to terms with her fear and discovers her own power in the process. He recognizes her ability to do this as 'both marvelous and courageous'. There is a clear prizing of Gina and her process—a warmth and admiration that is undeniable. He adds that 'it also fills me with enormous anger that we can't change the external situation'. Here we see more of the complexity of Carl's experience and Gina's impact on him—that he has also allowed himself to feel intense anger over the stupidity of a terrifying and needless situation existing in a 'world of intelligent people'. What is important to note is that neither of these strong feelings—the deep admiration and the intense anger—enter into Carl's reactions to Gina during the interview in any attempt to influence, change, diminish, or augment her experience or direction. He never breaks her direction by telling her he admires her, or by sharing his anger at the way things are. This is a very deep reflection of non-directivity. Though he may have experienced these feelings or impulses during the interview, he had the discipline to keep them out of the way—his responses appear to always follow Gina, not to follow his own internal frame or direction according to whatever emotions may arise within him. It is an ever present temptation in therapy to leave the client's frame for the comfort of the therapist's own frame; to reinforce the positive by expressing admiration, or perhaps to minimize something frightening or negative by changing the client's direction, pointing to the silver lining and avoiding the storm cloud. However, as well-intentioned as this type of therapist intervention may be at first glance, from the perspective of non-directive theory, it communicates conditions of worth. It may divert the client's attention from something fearful they are expressing, or communicate to them that they should not be feeling something that is intensely negative in some way. There is great potential in such statements to change or thwart the client's unique direction. Carl does not do this with Gina. He respects and values her as a true individual. In turn, she demonstrates an internal wisdom that enables her to find her own way.

NON-DIRECTIVITY AND THE POWER OF THE INDIVIDUAL

What is revolutionary, still, in Rogers' approach to psychotherapy, is the stance that no direction is needed from the therapist for the client to grow in a positive direction—the client is trusted completely in being the agent of change in her own life. The client has the capacity to change and grow, and will find her own pace and manner of doing what she needs to do. There is no emphasis on cure, in the sense of a resolution of symptoms through the application of a treatment by an 'expert' healer. From the standpoint of non-directivity, symptoms, so-called, may be seen as expressions of the client's efforts to be more fully herself in the face of conditions of worth imposed by others, as well as conditions of worth that are internally imposed. In other words, what may appear to be expressions of pathology are actually the seeds of some sort of growth, unfolding, or actualization. These seeds are always present, waiting to flourish in the right soil. The non-directive therapist trusts these expressions of the client's direction in all their forms, and has no need for, or interest in, diagnostic labels to categorize them for treatment. Such a non-directive perspective is not limited by the notion of cure, since there is always the potential for growth and movement beyond what otherwise might be considered cure.

This demonstration occurred over only twenty-eight exchanges between Gina and Carl, and was followed by a few observations made by each of them. Gina begins the interview with a tentative exploration of a fearful event in her life that she somehow feels stuck on.

Carl does not provide her with a cure for her fear or for her feeling stuck. He does not analyze her fear, reframe it, or search for cognitive underpinnings. He follows her direction. We do not see Gina coming away without fear. In fact, she is clear that the fear remains. What we do see is someone coming to a new place of awareness in relation to her fears. An awareness she has reached entirely in her own way. This new awareness leaves her feeling empowered, with a new relationship to her fear. As Rogers points out in the discussion segment, this is no mere passive acceptance of her fear. There is evidence of a deeper process that 'when one is at peace within oneself it is more possible to take effective social action'. Gina follows this with her own beautiful expression of self-awareness and growth: 'When I find that peace I get more power to do anything'. Ultimately, the power of non-directivity is centered within the emergent power of the individual.

REFERENCES

Brodley, BT (1999) The actualizing tendency concept in client-centered therapy. *The Person-Centered Journal, 6*, 108–20.

Bozarth, JD and Brodley, BT (1991) Actualisation: A functional concept in client-centered therapy. *Handbook of Self-Actualisation, 6*, 45–60.

Levitt, BE (2005) Non-directivity: The foundational attitude. In BE Levitt (ed) *Embracing Non-directivity: Reassessing person-centered theory and practice in the 21st century* (pp. 5–16). Ross-on-Wye: PCCS Books.

Raskin, NJ (1947/2005) The non-directive attitude. In BE Levitt (ed) *Embracing Non-directivity: Reassessing person-centered theory and practice in the 21st century* (pp. 5–16). Ross-on-Wye: PCCS Books.

Rogers CR (1942) *Counseling and Psychotherapy.* Cambridge, MA: Riverside Press.

Rogers, CR (1951) *Client-Centered Therapy: Its current practice, implication, and theory.* Boston: Houghton Mifflin.

Rogers, CR (1957) The necessary and sufficient conditions of personality change. *Journal of Consulting Psychology, 21*, 95–103.

Rogers, CR (1959) A theory of therapy, personality and interpersonal relationships, as developed in the client-centered framework. In S Koch (ed) *Psychology: A Study of a Science, Vol. 3, Formulations of the person and the social context* (pp. 184–256). New York: McGraw-Hill.

Rogers, CR (1963) The actualizing tendency in relation to 'motives' and to consciousness. In MR Jones (ed) *Nebraska Symposium on Motivation* (pp. 1–24). University of Nebraska Press.

Rogers CR (1983) *Gina*. Manuscript Division, Library of Congress, Washington, DC, Box 59/3.

CHAPTER 15

THE HALLUCINATION AS THE
UNCONSCIOUS SELF[1]

GARRY PROUTY

In the early 1990s, phenomenology was introduced into the field of psychiatry by the philosopher/psychiatrist Karl Jaspers (1963). This approach continued in Europe through such psychiatric writers as Binswanger (1963), Boss (1994), and Minkowski (1970). Major entry into the American psychotherapy literature was through the writings of Rollo May (1958). A brief historical review of existential-phenomenological psychiatry and psychotherapy is available in the literature (Halling and Dearborn, 1995).

Part of the phenomenological approach has been directed toward the schizophrenic hallucination (Boss, 1963; Laing, 1969; Strauss, 1966; Vandenberg, 1982). Carrying on with this tradition are the phenomenological articles of Prouty (1977, 1983, 1986, 1991), as well as Prouty and Pietrzak (1988). Those articles described methods of treatment as well as the lived experience of the hallucination. This paper attempts to describe an empathic,[2] experiential and process-oriented approach to the unconscious through the phenomenological medium of hallucinations.

The first clues as to the possibility of this emerged in actual hallucinatory work with psychotic clients (Prouty, 1994). One retarded/schizophrenic young man expressed his sense of the 'not yet conscious' in the following way:

> The evil thing is a picture. It's a purple picture that hangs there. It just hangs there and I can see it—the picture, you know. It's purple, it's very dark. So I can see it and I don't like it. I don't like it at all. It is very dark ... I don't like it at all. It's not good, this thing, whatever it is. *It's in the past* and it's very strong—the past—and it's over with and it's not coming back anymore. The

---

1. This chapter was first published in *The Journal of the American Academy of Psychoanalysis and Dynamic Psychiatry, 32,* 4, Winter, 2004, 598–612. New York: The Guilford Press.
2. Gallese's (2003) suggested non-reductionist model for empathy correlates the neural and phenomenological bases of intersubjectivity. He presents considerable empirical evidence for monkeys and humans that supports the concept of neural mechanisms that provide 'an implicit, automatic and unconscious' (p. 174) process of embodied simulation.
His hypothesis is that emotional sensitivity follows this same pattern of 'mirror neurons'. Phenomenologically he draws on the philosopher Husserl who postulates the body as the basis of conscious intersubjectivity. Continuing into the area of psychopathology, Gallese draws on phenomenological psychiatrists (Minkowski, Blankenberg and Paras) to formulate the view that schizophrenia is an empathic disorder, a failure in resonance with the world and with others.

past don't come back and this is like now. It ain't the *past*, you know. It's over with and I don't want to be tempted by it anymore. This thing, you know—has a very lot of strength to it. It's evil. You know. The thing has a very lot of strength to it. It's evil. It's no good and that's why it's no good at all. It's very evil, you know. I don't like it. It's very evil, this thing [pained laughter]. It's over with. It's *the past*, and it's not coming back anymore. (Prouty, 1994: 73-4. Emphasis added)

The client's emphasis on the past coming back is reported as a potentially imminent 'yet to be' experience. Perhaps something from the unconscious is beginning to emerge into consciousness?

THE PRE-SYMBOLIC THEORY OF HALLUCINATORY EXPERIENCE

THE PROBLEMATIC

Every conception has a starting point—a problematic (Peters, 1992; Prouty, Van Werde and Pörtner, 2001). In the case of hallucinations, the problematic is posed by Gendlin (1964), who described the hallucination as 'structure-bound'. This concept has several levels of meaning. First, hallucinations are perceived, literally, 'as such' and 'not his'. Next, the experiencing is considered isolated, meaning that the experiencing is not included in the felt functioning of the organism. Finally, this implicitly felt functioning is rigid—not in experiential process. Thus, Gendlin's concept of the hallucination can be described as a *non-process structure*. The problematic is how to turn this non-process structure into a process structure—from an hallucinatory image that does not process to an hallucinatory image that *does* process, according to experiential principles.

THE PHILOSOPHICAL PRIMACY OF THE SYMBOL

The philosophical primacy of the symbol refers to an epistemological shift from *experiencing* to the *symbolizing of experience*. This philosophical primacy of the symbol is asserted by Cassirer (1955), who described the human as 'Animal Symbolicum'. This philosophical impulse is further expanded by Susan Langer (1961), who described the human brain as a 'transformer'. The brain transforms 'the current of experience into symbols'. This philosophical focus allows us to think of humankind as 'motivated' to symbolize experience. This philosophical emphasis on symbolization is perhaps best represented in psychoanalysis by Kubie (1953) and Searles (1965), who both saw this capacity as the unique hallmark of humans.

170

THE SEMIOTICS OF ABSTRACTNESS—CONCRETENESS

These insights, however, do not produce semiotic conceptualizations about different levels of symbolization. Reichenbach (cited in Szasz, 1961) conceived such a semiotic conceptualization as levels of abstraction and concreteness. The most abstract form of symbolizing experience is the *meta-symbol*. It does not directly refer to an experience, but to a set of processes beyond direct experience. An example of a *meta-symbol* is E = MC^2. This process cannot be directly experienced. The next level of symbolizing experience is called *object-language*. This refers to everyday ordinary cultural speech, such as book, chair and so forth. Continuing to a more concrete level, Reichenbach describes the *indexical-sign*. This symbolization is a concrete experience that refers to a concrete experience; for example, cloud can refer to rain, or snow can refer to cold. Next in the continuum of concreteness is the *iconical-sign*. This is a literal duplicate of the referent; a photograph or TV image, for example. An even more primitive form of concreteness is called the *pre-symbol* (Prouty, 1986). Drawing conceptualizations from Jaspers, the pre-symbol can be described in the following way: 'It cannot be clarified by someone else' and 'it is inseparable from what it symbolizes' (Jaspers, 1971: 124).

INTRODUCING THE PRE-SYMBOL

The term *pre-symbol* refers to the structure of the hallucinatory image as distinct from its processing. Psychotherapy with hallucinatory images reveals that the images contain two properties—one phenomenological and the other symbolic. This creates a definitional polarity.
1. Sartre (1956) defines the phenomenon as an experience that is 'absolutely self-indicative'. This means an experience indicates itself, refers to itself, or means itself.
2. Whitehead (1927) describes symbol as 'an experience that indicates another experience' (p. 8). Symbols are experiences that mean or refer to other experiences.

Expressed in another way, the phenomenon is 'about itself', and the symbol is 'about something else'. These two polarities require a synthesis to describe fully the structure of the hallucination. This necessitates conceptualizing the pre-symbol.

STRUCTURAL PROPERTIES OF THE PRE-SYMBOL

Expressive
As an expressive structure, the hallucination is described as 'self-intentional'. As already mentioned, Langer (1961) viewed the human brain as something that transforms the current of experience into symbols. This metaphor allows us to think of the hallucination as an expressive transformation of real-life experience into image-form. One patient described this self-intentionality by saying, 'These images are my unconscious trying to express itself'. Another patient described it as, 'the past trying to come back'. Still another conveyed the volitional quality by saying, 'The images start in my unconscious and move towards my consciousness to be real'.

Phenomenological

As an experiential structure, the hallucinatory image is described as 'self-indicating'. It is experienced as real, and as such it implies itself. Experience A implies Experience A. The hallucination means *itself as itself.* Exemplifying this, one schizophrenic patient said, 'it's real, it is … it's very real … I see it … over there … It makes sounds too'.

Symbolic

As a symbolic structure, the hallucination is described as 'self-referential'. It is an experience that implies another experience. Experience A implies Experience B. The hallucinatory image (Experience A) contains its referent (Experience B) within itself. The hallucinatory image means *itself within itself.* A case example is that an hallucinatory python (Experience A) experientially processes into a real homicidal mother (Experience B). The python functions as a symbol of the mother.

HALLUCINATORY PROCESS

The following vignette (Prouty, 1991) shows how pre-symbolic experiencing is deeply rooted in the phenomenological approach and illustrates the self-intentional, self-indicating and self-referential properties of the hallucinations.

> The patient, a male aged nineteen, was diagnosed as moderately retarded (Stanford Binet IQ of 65). He was from upper lower class origin of Polish ethnicity. There was no mental illness in the family, and the client had not been diagnosed or treated for mental illness: that is, he was not receiving any medications for psychosis. He was a day-client in a vocational rehabilitation workshop for the mentally retarded. He was referred to me for therapy because of his severe withdrawal and non-communication. The patient also behaved as though he was very frightened. He was shaking and trembling at his workstation and during his bus ride to the facility. At home, he rarely talked with his parents and he never socialized with neighborhood peers.
>
> During the early phases of therapy, the patient expressed almost nothing and made very little contact with me. He was very frightened during the sessions and could barely tolerate being in the room with me. Gradually, with the aid of contact reflections, the client accepted a minimal relationship and expressed himself in a minimal way. Eventually, it became clear, the patient was terrorized by hallucinations that were constantly present to him.
>
> The following description provides an account of pre-symbolic experiencing. It provides an outline of hallucinatory movement and its subsequent resolution about its origin.

Phase I: 'The purple demon'
Client: It's very evil, this thing. What it wants to do is to rip me apart, you know. It's very evil … and it's very evil, this thing. That's why I don't want anything to do with it. I'm tempted by it, you know. It's so small but it has so much strength and it wants to rip me

172

apart, you know. It wants to drive me into the past. It wants … it wants to make the past come back and I don't want the past to come back like it did a long time ago. It's over with, you know. It's not coming back anymore. The past doesn't come back. It's over with already.

Therapist: It's evil and strong. It wants the past to come back.

C: The evil thing is a picture. It's a purple picture that hangs there. It just hangs and I can see it. I can see it … the picture, you know. It's purple, it's very dark. It's very dark. So I can see it and I don't like it at all. It's very dark.

T: It's a dark purple picture and you don't like it.

C: And it's very tempted and I don't want to be tempted by it. It's very small. It's very evil, you know … that's all … It just hangs there. It don't do nothing. It's very evil, you know. It's just like a picture. A purple picture. It just stays there. It just stays there, you know … the picture. It don't do nothing. It's evil, you know. I don't like it at all. It's not good and this thing, whatever it is. It's in the past and it's very strong, the past. … And it's over with and I don't want to be tempted by it any more. Yeh, yeh, it's very evil, very evil and very strong and has a lot of strength to it.

T: It's evil and it's in the past. It's strong and it hangs there. You don't want to be tempted by it.

C: This thing, you know … this thing has a lot of strength to it. It's evil, you know … This thing has a lot of strength to it. It's evil. It's not good and that's why it's very evil, this thing. [Pained laughter.]
It's over with. It's in the past, and it's not coming back anymore. It's over with a long time ago, you know. It's not going to come back anymore. I used to talk about the trees and the flowers, grass, and its all over with. It's not coming back anymore. It's something else, the picture. The purple picture just hangs there. It's evil. No?

T: The purple picture just hangs there. It's evil and you don't like it.

C: The past, it came from the past and the past is over with. It's not coming back any more, you know.

T: It comes from the past.

C: It's a picture. It's just a picture. A big, purple picture. It just hangs there. I don't think it will rip me apart. I think it's very strong, but it ain't going to rip me apart. I don't think it will rip me apart at all, no.

T: It's a big, purple picture. It won't rip you apart.

173

C: The thing is getting big and large. It's very big and large. It wants to get me. I won't let it. It's evil. It's like a demon, a bad demon. It wants to chop me all up. I won't let it chop me all up because it's bad. Very bad.
[Loud sobs.]
Just a temptation, like any other temptation. A temptation is a temptation. You shouldn't be tempted by it and you know I want to pull away from it. I don't want to go by it.

T: It's big and large and evil. It wants to chop you. It's very tempting.

C: It's very bad and it's very destructive. It ain't good at all by it. It's like a bad demon, like a ... like a demon or evil or something. Like a demon devil and I don't care for it too much. You know, at all. I ... I don't like it too much, no. I don't like it at all, this thing. It's very bad and very evil, you know. It ain't no good. It's very bad. It's with the past and its not going to come back any more. It's over with, you know, and talking about the trees and flowers and grass, and that's over. I mean it's not coming back, but this is right now, I mean.

T: It's bad and destructive, like an evil demon. It's evil and in the past.

C: It's not coming back, but this is right here now. I can feel it, you know. It's like air. It's up above me. It's very close up above and I can feel ... almost touch it, you know. It's so close, very close. It's like a demon, you know, demon devil or something. 'Ho, ho, hoing' and all like that, you know ... very bad, very bad. It forces me, pressing, very pressing on me ... it's very pressing, it forces, a lot of force to it and it wants to grab me, you know. It wants to grab me. The feeling wants to grab me. The feeling wants to grab me.

T: It's very close and it wants to grab you.

C: The feeling ... the feeling ... ah, it's in the picture. The feeling is in the picture. Yes, it's there and I can see it. I don't like it. It's over with, you know. It's like the past and it's not coming back any more. It's over. It's just the trees and the flowers and grass and that's over and it's not coming back.

Phase 1 describes a purple demonic image that just 'hangs there'. The patient experiences it as evil and powerful. The image is considered destructive and wants to rip the patient apart. This phase contains the property of being self-intentional. The patient expresses: 'It wants to drive me into the past. It wants to make the past come back and I don't want the past to come back the way it did a long time ago ... It's over with, you know ... it's not coming back anymore ... already ... It's in the past and it's very strong, the past, and its over with and it's not coming back any more'. As illustrated by this example, self-intentional means the expressive transformation of real-life experiences into images.

Phase II: 'Orange square hate'

C: *It's orange, the color's in a square. It's an orange color that's square. It's an orange color that's square and it hates me. And it don't even like me. It hates me.*

T: *It's orange and it's square and it hates you.*

C: *It hates me a lot, you know, and it scares me. I get scared because of that. I get scared because it hates me.*

T: *It's orange and it's square and you get scared a lot.*

C: *And because it's orange that scares me and I get scared of the bad hating.*

T: *The orange and bad hating scare you a lot. That hate scares you.*

C: *I get scared because of that. I get scared a lot. I get scared of the orange thing. It's orange.*

T: *You get scared of the orange thing.*

C: *Big orange, square thing. It's square and it's orange and I hate it. It don't like me because it hates me. It hates me and I get scared and I get excited over it too. I get very excited.*

T: *You get very excited.*

C: *It's exciting; I get excited over it too. I do. I do. I get excited over it a lot. What? I get scared a lot about it. It makes noises. It makes noises.*

T: *It's orange and it makes noises.*

C: *It makes noises . . . It hates me. It also gets very excited. It gets very excited. It does, it gets me very excited a lot. I get, I get, I get very excited over it. I do. I do. I do. There's so much hate and it scares me and it makes me uncomfortable. It does. And it's real . . . It's real, it is.*

T: *It's real.*

C: *It is, it's very real.*

T: *It's very real . . . You point to it. It's over on your side. You see it.*

C: *I see it. Over there. Over there.*

T: It's over there.

C: It makes sounds too.

Phase II has an image that is orange, square and has hate in it. The patient is very frightened of it. Phase II contains self-indicating properties because it is experienced as real, as a phenomenon. It implies itself. The patient's process is as follows: 'and it's real, it is … It is, it's very real … I see it … Over there. Over there … It makes a sound, too.'

Phase III: 'Mean lady'
C: Yeah, well. Yeah, I would. I would. She's … I don't know. There we go. What? What?
[Auditory hallucination.]

T: OK. Let's talk about what you see.

C: Well, it ain't real, you know, and she ain't real, you know. What?
[Auditory hallucination.]
Ha, ha, ha.
[Sobs.]
She has orange hair and yellow eyes.

T: She has orange hair and yellow eyes.

C: She's very pretty. She's very pretty. She loves getting mean when I am bad. She could get … she's mean, you know.

T: She's pretty and mean.

C: She is. She is. No, really she is. Really she is, with yellow eyes and orange hair. Boy! That scares me. That scares me a lot. That scares me a lot … Yeah, both the meanness and the … What?
[Auditory hallucination.]
Yeah. Aah. I can see it and I don't even want to see it. It's over with and it's not coming back any more. And I can see it.

T: You can see it.

C: Yeah, that scares me. Yeah, it does. I think about it. It scares me.

T: When you think about it, that scares you.

C: I get scared. I don't want to think about it. I got it. I got it.

T: You don't want to think about it but you got it.

C: I got it. It's orange, you know. That's helping. She's helping.

T: She's helping.

C: She scares me, though, she scares me. But as long as I'm good, as long as I'm good, I am ... she's a friend.

T: As long as you're good, she's a friend.

C: But she's scary.

T: She's scary.

C: Scary. Yellow eyes, orange hair she has, she does. Reminds me of a dragon, you know. Her eyes are like that.

T: Her eyes are like a dragon.

C: Almost, you know, like a dragon ... Her eyes are like a dragon ... She's strong ... She's strong, I'm weak. And I'm good, but she's also mean. She can be mean too, see? And I'm good if I'm good and I am, I really am, but she's all ... she's very mean. She can be mean ... and it scares me.

T: She's mean and that scares you.

C: She looks over me. She watches over me, but she has eyes like a dragon ... Right. That's like a dragon and then she scares me and I get scared.

At this point, the patient appeared upset and wanted the tape recorder turned off. Over the next two sessions, the image processed into a nun who had beaten the retarded client because he did not understand his school lessons.

Phase III contains an image of a woman that the patient describes as pretty, mean and scary. She has orange hair and yellow eyes. This deeply frightens the patient. The significant theoretical observation of this phase is its processing to its experience of origin. The patient recaptures a real memory of being beaten by a nun who punished him for not completing his school lessons. This phase illustrates the self-referential property of hallucinations; that is, it symbolizes an experience within itself. It refers to an 'originating' event (the nun).

THE NEWER THEORETICAL FINDINGS

The following observations can be made concerning the particular case: (1) The hallucinatory structure can be processed through to an unconscious level; (2) the meaning of the hallucination can be integrated; and (3) hallucinatory processing leads to a realistic and traumatic etiology. Numerous other case histories detail the pre-symbolic processing of hallucinatory images (Boss, 1963; Prouty, 1977, 1983, 1986, 1991; Prouty and Pietrzak, 1988); these reveal insights concerning such issues as the structure of primary process and the structure of the schizophrenic self. Romme and Escher (1993) describe therapy for hallucinatory voices utilizing support groups.

PRIMARY PROCESS

Freud included both the dream and the hallucination in his concept of primary process. Assigning such limited value to consciousness, Freud paid little or no attention to the phenomenology of consciousness being developed by the philosopher Husserl. This is interesting because both were students of the philosopher Brentano. If one compares the phenomenology of dreams with the phenomenology of hallucinations, it is easy to see 'the dream is my dream' and 'I had it last night'. It is something experienced, which plays itself out within the boundaries of self, and is a memory. The hallucination is disconnected: it becomes experienced as not belonging to the self, but rather as an external reality that is immediate. Therefore, in contrast to a dream, which Freud labeled a 'projection' (within the self boundary—mine, internal etc.), I describe the hallucination as an 'extrojection' (outside of the self boundary—not mine, external etc.). On the basis of this phenomenological distinction, the dream is labeled 'projection', whereas the hallucination can be termed 'extrojection'.

A DIVIDED SELF

Polster and Polster (1974), from the perspective of gestalt psychotherapy, describe the dream as a fragment of the self. It is simple to extrapolate this perspective to understanding the hallucination. The hallucination is a self-fragment split off from the self-structure— a severe rupture in the fabric of self. This presents a picture close to RD Laing's (1969) description of the 'Divided Self'—to borrow his famed title. Schizophrenia, thus, can be partially described as a severe split in the self-structure. The psychotherapy of hallucinations therefore leads to re-integration of self in schizophrenia. Many years ago, I used to see state hospital schizophrenics wandering the wards speaking and gesticulating towards 'empty' space. I now see these patients as relating to fragments of the self that contain the potentiality for re-integration. Perhaps Laing's (1969: 71) concept of the 'unembodied self' captures this picture.

THE UNCONSCIOUS

Freud described the dream as the 'Royal Road to the Unconscious'; the hallucination is also a 'Royal Road to the Unconscious'. There is an important distinction, however. Freud's data from his original inference of the unconscious were dreams, hypnosis and slips of the tongue (Boss, 1994), whereas the original datum for the description of the unconscious is the client's hallucinatory experience. This emphasis on direct experience must be considered in contrast with the psychoanalytic view of Nunberg (1955) who states *we possess no direct evidence of the existence of the unconscious. We deduce it from indirect evidence* (p. 6, emphasis added).

The use of an experiential hallucinatory method to approach the unconscious is predicated on several grounds. The first is accessibility. The hallucination can present itself as an immediacy to consciousness (now), whereas the dream is a past memory (last night). Closely linked to accessibility is the issue of experiential presence. Hallucinations can be well-lighted, multicolored and available for years (Havens, 1962). Their next experiential value is their capacity to be processed to their realistic origins. Finally, the hallucinatory image itself can be thought of as an experiential fragment of the unconscious, thereby providing a direct approach.

A SPATIAL PHENOMENOLOGY OF THE UNCONSCIOUS

McCall (1983), quoting the views of Heidegger, described phenomenological hermeneutics in the following manner: 'Hermeneutics is a method of *uncovering* (*unverborgen*), of remaining with the experience until it reveals its hidden truth' (p. 113). The following psychiatric description fulfills, I hope, this definition.

Medard Boss (1963) entitled a chapter of his book 'A patient who taught the author to think differently'. It is in this spirit that the evidence of a three-dimensional phenomenology of the unconscious is presented. Ellenberger (1958) outlined the various theoretical contributions to the phenomenology of spatiality. However, none of these is concerned with the hallucination per se.

The patient was a woman in her forties who was schizophrenic, homicidal/suicidal, as well as abusive of alcohol. The total length of treatment was nine years. Ten years later, the client and I spent a long time tape recording and preparing manuscripts about the therapeutic process (Prouty, 2000). In the course of the therapy, the patient had an intense hallucination of a python experientially processed to a homicidal mother (Prouty, 1994). Also, a number of smaller and less intense hallucinations were processed. In the original treatment, these hallucinations had been presented sequentially by the patient. The interesting new observation was that the therapist never realized these hallucinations were present in three-dimensional space, commingled with the patient's reality perception: they were all present at the same time. They were experienced as a unified spatial gestalt. Perhaps analogously, they could be seen as parallel to having several dreams at the same time in a single reality space.

The patient experienced eight hallucinations at the same continuing time, within real space. A realistic description is as follows: first there was a python curled in front of the table between the patient's and the therapist's chairs. This, resolved with treatment (Prouty, 1983), represented her mother's homicidal 'agent'. Concurrently, between the python and the table-lamp, appeared Sonja in an ephemeral form. The patient described her as a siren, seducing the client towards suicidal death, repeating, 'Peace, Peace'. Sonja was a tactile hallucination, and the client integrated her meaning through inserting her arm into her ephemeral body and experiencing warm 'intestine-like' sensations. The patient experienced this as disgusting, repulsive and nauseating. Sonja was also a murderous 'agent' (patient's language) for the patient's homicidal mother.

Also concurrently, another negative figure, a dwarf, was named 'The Judge'. He rendered death sentences for very minor infractions; for example, losing a rubber band. The patient described him as a 'hanging judge' who would declare her worthless, deserving to die, and so forth. He would yell 'off with her head' and 'she is guilty ... guilty ... guilty'. Again he was an 'agent' of the homicidal mother. Finally, and simultaneously, the Tasmanian Devil was a tornado-like, swirling dervish with sharp teeth. In therapy, the patient described it as her mother's chaotic anger.

At the same time, slightly behind the patient's chair and left shoulder, appeared Marie, the abused child. She was imprisoned and isolated behind bars. The child was the same age as the patient's murdered friend. Also at this age, the patient was locked in the refrigerator by the patient's homicidal mother. Further, the hallucinated child was the same age as the patient when she was sent to the darkened basement, by her homicidal mother, while a real murderer was in the neighborhood. Marie was 'healed' by the appearance of a kitten who became her best 'friend'. To this day, the client has close relationships with pet cats. In fact, she has one deceased cat preserved by a taxidermist.

There were also several 'positive' figures. Behind the therapist's chair appeared a more positive apparition called Gus. Gus was a quietly spoken, Thoreau-like fisherman, who was a gentle, down-to-earth, wise, intelligent and helpful figure. One is reminded of Jung's 'wise old man' archetype. Two young boys, like (Huck Finn and Tom Sawyer) finished the roster of the patient's spatial hallucinations. She reported that the boys felt like 'innocence'.

After the intensive experiential treatment of the python was finished (Prouty, 1983), a new, ninth image appeared. The image was of the patient's mother with the python crawling back into her breasts. Instantly, with clarity, the patient realized her mother's homicidal intent. The gestalt unity of hallucinations immediately lost its emotional intensity and passed away, presenting a normal spatiality for the office.

DISCUSSION

It is important to understand that this was a three-dimensional network of images that contained positive and negative unconscious content. Three of the pathogenic images (Python, Sonja and Judge) were co-functioning as agents of the homicidal mother. This was an organized gestalt through which therapeutic processing of hallucinations enabled direct experiential access to unconscious material (the homicidal mother). The next very important observation is that the content of the unconscious, thus far, has appeared as realistic trauma, as well as other experiential potentials of the personality, both positive and negative (Mahrer, 1996). When the hallucinatory content was integrated or became conscious, the hallucinatory self-fragment contained the unconscious. Thus, we may speak of the hallucination as a fragment of the unconscious.

CONCLUSION

This chapter has explored the psychotic hallucination from a symbolic and experiential perspective. Starting from Gendlin's (1964) conception of the hallucination as 'structure-bound' experiencing, the problem is formulated as how to develop the hallucination into process experiencing. The first step is a philosophical shift from a purely phenomenological assumption (the human is experiential) to a symbolic assumption (the human symbolizes experience). The symbolizing of experience is presented on a continuum of abstractness/concreteness ending with the pre-symbol, 'which cannot be clarified by something else' and 'is inseparable from what it symbolizes'. In phenomenological terms the pre-symbol is described as 'self-indicative' and in symbolical terms as 'self-referential', while the motivation to symbolize experience is described as 'self-intentional'. In addition to concrete illustrations, the case material demonstrates these concepts in the therapeutic-experiential process of hallucinations.

Two aspects of schizophrenia were explored: (a) primary process and (b) the divided self. Freud described dreams and hallucinations as one concept—primary process. Failing to use phenomenology, Freud did not identify significant differences between them. The dream is something experienced within the boundary of the self; the hallucination is experienced as not within the boundary of the self. This phenomenological distinction suggests a different language of description. The dream is a 'projection' within the experiential boundaries of the self, and the hallucination is an 'extrojection' outside the experiential boundaries of the self.

Laing's famed book title *The Divided Self* (1969) finds clinical affirmation in that the hallucinatory self-fragment is severely dissociated or split off from the core self. The result, a partial understanding of schizophrenia as a profound rending of the self-structure, casts psychotherapy in the role of integrating the self-fragment into the core self.

One fundamental issue explored concerns the conceptualization of the unconscious. As described by Freud, the unconscious is an 'inference' from experience: for example, dreams, slips of the tongue and hypnosis. The unconscious as described in this paper is not an inference; it is a direct manifestation derived from the hallucinatory experiencing and processing. Perhaps it is best expressed as the 'not-conscious'.

The same case study of the clinical processing of hallucinations with a chronic schizophrenic woman revealed a spatial phenomenology that included multiple hallucinations, perhaps like several dreams within the same reality space at the same time. Her hallucinations proved capable of experiential processing to unconscious content. Because the hallucinations were fragments of the self that contained unconscious experience, it is consistent to describe hallucinations as the unconscious self. The spatial gestalt of the several hallucinations thus provides us with a spatial phenomenology for the client's unconscious.

REFERENCES

Binswanger, L (1963) Introduction to schizophrenia. In L Binswanger *Being-in-the-World* (pp. 241–63). New York: Basic Books.

Boss, M (1963) A patient who taught the author to see and think differently. In M Boss, *Psychoanalysis and Daseinanalysis* (pp. 5–27). New York: Basic Books.

Boss, M (1994) *Existential Foundations of Medicine and Psychology*. London: Jason Aronson.

Cassirer, E (1955) Man—an animal symbolicum. In D Dunes (ed) *Treasury of Philosophy* (pp. 227–9). New York: Philosophical Library.

Ellenberger, E (1958) Psychiatric phenomenology and existential Analysis. In R May (ed) *Existence: A new dimension in psychiatry and psychology* (pp. 108–14). New York: Basic Books.

Gallese, V (2003) The roots of empathy: The shared manifold and the neural basis of inter-subjectivity. *Psychopathology, 36,* 171–80.

Gendlin, ET (1964) A theory of personality change. In P Worschel and D Byrne (eds) *Personality Change* (pp. 102–48). New York: John Wiley.

Halling, S and Dearborn, J (1995) A brief history of existential phenomenological psychiatry and psychotherapy. *Journal of Phenomenological Psychology, 26,* 1–45.

Havens, L (1962) The placement and movement of hallucinations in space: Phenomenology and theory. *International Journal of Psychoanalysis, 43,* 426–35.

Jaspers, K (1963) The subjective phenomenon of morbid psychic life. In *General Psychopathology* (p. 55). Chicago: University of Chicago Press.

Jaspers, K (1971) *Philosophy, 3.* Chicago: University of Chicago Press.

Kubie, L (1953) The distortion of the symbolic process in neurosis and psychosis. *Journal of the American Psychoanalytical Association, 1,* 57–83.

Laing, RD (1969) *The Divided Self.* New York: Pantheon Books.

Langer, S (1961) *Philosophy in a New Key.* New York: Mentor Books.

Mahrer, A (1996) *The Complete Guide to Experiential Psychotherapy.* New York: John Wiley.

May, R (1958) *Existence: A new dimension in psychology and psychiatry.* New York: Basic Books.

McCall, RJ (1983) *Phenomenological Psychology.* Madison: University of Wisconsin Press.

Minkowski, E (1970) Schizophrenia. *Lived Time: Phenomenological and psychopathological studies* (pp. 272–89). Evanston: Northwestern Universities Press.

Nunberg, H (1955) *Principles of Psychoanalysis: Their application to the neuroses.* New York: International Universities Press.

Peters, H (1992) *Psychotherapie bij geestelijk gehandicapten.* Amsterdam: Swets and Zeitlinger.

Polster, E and Polster, M (1974) *Gestalt Therapy Integrated.* New York: Vintage Books.

Prouty, GF (1977) Protosymbolic method: A phenomenological treatment of schizophrenics. *International Journal of Mental Imagery, 1,* 339–42.

Prouty, GF (1983) Hallucinatory contact: A phenomenological treatment of schizophrenics. *Journal of Communication Therapy, 2,* 99–103.

Prouty, GF (1986) The pre-symbolic structure and therapeutic transformation of hallucinations. In M Wolpin, J Schorr and L Kreuger (eds) *Imagery, Vol. 4* (pp. 99–106). New York: Plenum Press.

Prouty, GF (1991) The pre-symbolic structure and processing of schizophrenic hallucinations. In L Fusek (ed) *New Directions in Client-Centered Therapy: Practice with difficult practice populations* (pp. 1–18). Chicago: Chicago Counseling, Psychotherapy and Research Center.

Prouty, GF (1994) *Theoretical Evolutions in Person-Centered/Experiential Therapy: Applications to schizophrenic and retarded psychoses.* Welport, CT: Praeger.

Prouty, GF (2000) Courage and self-actualization. Unpublished manuscript.

Prouty, GF and Pietrzak, S (1988) Pre-Therapy method applied to persons experiencing hallucinatory images. *Person-Centered Review, 3,* 426–41.

Prouty, GF, Van Werde, D and Pörtner, M (2001) *Pre-therapie.* Maarssen, The Netherlands: Elsiever.

Prouty, GF, Van Werde, D and Pörtner, M (2002) *Pre-Therapy.* Ross-on-Wye: PCCS Books.

Romme, M and Escher, S (1993) *Accepting Voices.* London: Mind Publications.

Sartre, J-P (1956) *Being and Nothingness.* New York: Washington Square Press.

Searles, H (1965) The differentiation between concrete and metaphorical thinking in the recovering schizophrenic. *Collected Papers on Schizophrenia and Related Subjects* (pp. 560–1). London: Hogarth Press.

Strauss, E (1966) Phenomenology and hallucinations. *Phenomenological Psychology* (pp. 277–87). New York: Basic Books.

Szasz, T (1961) *The Myth of Mental Illness.* New York: Hoeber-Harper.

Vandenberg, J (1982) On hallucinating: Critical-historical overview and guidelines for further study. In J De Koning and F Jenner (eds) *Phenomenological Psychiatry* (pp. 97–110). New York: Academic Press, Grune and Stratton.

Whitehead, AN (1927) *Symbolism.* New York: Capricorn Books.

CHAPTER 16

IN PLACE OF THE MEDICAL MODEL: PERSON-CENTRED ALTERNATIVES TO THE MEDICALISATION OF DISTRESS

PETE SANDERS

INTRODUCTION

Distress is a part of everyday life. It covers a very wide range of experiences from the trivial to the overwhelming and enduring, with none immune from its effects. In Chapter 3 of *Person-Centred Psychopathology: A positive psychology of mental health* I argued that thinking in terms of mental *illness* instead of moderate to severe psychological *distress* is outdated, and runs against both person-centred theory and current evidence. Having made that argument it is reasonable to ask what I propose in place of the medical model of mental illness with all of its attendant structures, services and treatments. In this chapter I sketch one possible alternative—informed by my involvement with the person-centred approach (PCA) for almost 35 years—to the picture painted by medical model of mental illness.

It is argued that the Western medical model of mental illness has improved the lives of countless people, particularly since the advent of neuroleptic medication in the 1950s. However, there is evidence to dispute this widely held view. Recovery rates from schizophrenia over the long term have not improved in the past fifty years (Harding et al., 1987; Harding and Zahnister,1994; Sargent, 1966). More reasons why I and many others are not satisfied and call for change can be found, for example, in Sanders (2005, 2006b, 2007), Read, Mosher and Bentall (2004) and Maddux, Snyder and Lopez (2004).

The 'model' at the centre of this alternative way of thinking and acting is that distress is most frequently the result of complex events in the environments in which we live and our reactions to them, mediated by our predispositions both psychological and biological.[1] This is not a new idea. However, there is no single convenient answer to the important question of how to think about distress and help people in distress. Instead of a simple answer—no matter how badly we might wish for one—what we find is a series of debates between the many stakeholders whose voices demand to be heard. I say 'stakeholders' because distressed people (service users), carers, friends, family, doctors, psychologists, psychiatrists, scientists in drug companies, therapists, indeed all citizens,

---

1. Social models and other alternatives to biological psychiatry and the medical model do not dispute that a person's biology may dispose them to react in a particular way to stress. They do not, however, start and finish with biology as the only, or primary, explanation. In a social model, biology assumes its evidenced weighting alongside material, social and psychological factors. The evidence is a matter of dispute.

have a stake in how our society understands and deals with distress. It is simultaneously big business and intimately personal, and many things in between. Someone's stake in distress (including my own), whether commercial, professional or personal, has the potential to influence their experience and judgement.

This sketch of a model can be considered to have as much authority as any done on the back of a cigarette packet in a pub; as much, if not more, inherent logic as the medical model and a lot less sponsorship from drug companies. But do not underestimate the authority, commonsense and purchasing power of the citizen, for it is as one I speak now, albeit with more structural power and differently informed, as a consequence of my professional roles over the years, than most. But a citizen none the less—someone whose life (and the lives of those close to me) has been, and could again be affected any day by severe distress. This chapter is a call to all like-minded citizens to make their voices heard. And international public opinion is on our side. Read and Haslam (2004) reviewed research in nine countries on 'mental health literacy' and public opinion on medical interventions, finding that the public prefers psychosocial explanations and solutions to distress over medical ones.

The professionals involved in helping distressed people (psychiatrists, psychologists and psychotherapists), are themselves caught in the same flow of complex and often conflicting demands and information—the demands of politicians and the media; the needs of carers and distressed people; the seductive illusion of a chemical panacea; the need for drug companies to remain profitable. The professional's *job*, however, is to interpret this in everyone's service, so that the best solutions are available to as many people as possible. At the same time they have more to lose than other stakeholders in terms of power, influence and earnings—which might help us understand their resistance to change. This is why we must make sure that the evidence they review is wide-ranging, includes 'experts by experience' (distressed people and carers), and is impartially collected and evaluated so that no single group of stakeholders is privileged, save possibly distressed people themselves.

The tendency towards the biologisation of experience and the medicalisation of distress insidiously causes us to think in reductionistic, compartmentalised ways. We are encouraged to think of humanness in terms of brain structure, chemicals and genes, independent of the relations within ourselves, between each other and the world. We are encouraged to think of human flourishing in terms of 'health' and 'illness'. This is, as Dave Mearns (2006) points out, a 'deficiency' model of humanity, not a 'potentiality' model, or an approach which can speak to the positive side of human experience (Seligman, 2003). Such a deficiency model of being human requires the individual getting the right 'doses' of things, from essential fats to Mozart, in order to be made whole. The PCA and *social* models[2] do not compartmentalise or reduce human living to doses of approved substances and experiences. We should, therefore, not be persuaded into thinking that the collecting of evidence must mimic that which is appropriate for

---

2. Readers wishing to read more about social models are advised to visit the Social Perspectives Network website: <http://www.spn.org.uk>.

'doses' of drugs—the so-called 'gold standard' of randomised controlled trials (RCT). Human relationships cannot be measured into approved therapeutic 'doses', regardless of the time-limited propaganda put out by medical economists.

But before I move on, I must consider whether this chapter, in a book of case studies, should be a case study of what a person-centred social model of distress might look like, or a case study of what professional and social action we might all take to supplant the medical model of mental illness with a social model of distress.

I have tried to make it a starter in both, but quite deliberately, indeed tactically, incomplete. No *one* person, nor group of people, whether they be professionals, carers or currently distressed people, should have the monopoly on determining the methodology of understanding and responding to distress. The new way of thinking must start with a new methodology for its own genesis; we must all commit to a multidisciplinary and multifactorial process without knowing where it will end, save the pre-condition that no single group shall be the guardians of the metaphor.

METAPHOR REASSIGNMENT

The idea that distress is an illness, is just that, an idea. It is, as many have pointed out over the years, simply a codification of ordinary judgments about madness with no scientific value (Pilgrim and Rogers, 2005; Coulter, 1973; Bentall, 1990; Boyle, 1999, 2002; Maddux, Snyder, and Lopez, 2004). Or, according to Wing (1978), psychological 'disorders' are names for theories, not names for things that exist in nature. It is a metaphor for how things look and feel when people are distressed.

'Illness' has been used as a metaphor for a lot of things that, with hindsight, we no longer think of as being illnesses. The metaphors have been *reassigned* over the years, some within my lifetime. For example, many of my friends ceased to be ill in 1973 on the day that 'homosexuality' was taken out of the American Psychiatric Association's *Diagnostic and Statistical Manual for Mental Disorders* (*DSM*). The women's movement struggled, and has at least in part succeeded, to remove pregnancy and menstruation from the list of 'pathologies' associated with simply being a woman. Disability is no longer seen as a medical condition per se—disabled people may be different, but they are not *ill*. There has been a shift, however small in some cases, from being '*patients* without knowledge' to being '*persons* with knowledge' (Madigan, 1999) and in these domains of life, knowledge is indeed power.

These examples of widely held illness metaphors which have changed in the past fifty years assure readers that this is not a lost cause. Many people think that the 'psychiatric system' is too big, has too many political connections or has too much inertia to make change possible. Nevertheless, I believe the signs are there to suggest that soon it will be the time to change our ideas that distress is an illness like any other, and helping professionals must stand up alongside service users to dismantle the metaphor.

The above metaphor reassignments did not happen as a result of wishful thinking, but after much suffering, campaigning and social action by the victims of the oppressive and inappropriate metaphor and their supporters. Similarly, and for a number of reasons, the medical model will not yield to a different metaphor without a struggle. Metaphors are often maintained beyond the point at which they hold the best interests of the majority of stakeholders (in this case the users of mental health services, their carers, friends and families) because of past progress, current powerful vested interests, inertia and the pain of change. Although the medical model has provided (and continues to provide) comfort for many, just as it did with the medicalisation of disability, pregnancy, sexuality, etc., there comes a point at which progress becomes arrested, and the metaphor begins to stagnate thinking and distort action. It soon becomes increasingly likely that change is possible towards a new way of understanding which will serve the interests of the majority of stakeholders better. It might even be achieved without a bloody revolution if a viable alternative can at least be imagined. We can then start the serious business of organised social action and talking it into being. I am guessing that such a moment is imminent with regard to the illness metaphor of distress—so I'm talking.

It is often the case in the difficult domains of human social behaviour (anti-social behaviour, public nuisance, crime) that we would rather not engage with the problems in person, but pay someone else such as the police or social workers to do the unpleasant work for us. And so it is with distress, since people in distress are sometimes distressing to have around. Distress is distressing to witness because it is both an inconvenient interruption to the otherwise smooth running of my life and a constant reminder of my own vulnerability. I would much rather be able to phone for people in white coats to take away the person behaving oddly in the high street or railway carriage, safe in the belief that it has nothing to do with me. My own comfort helps keep the medical model in its dominant position against the huge weight of evidence, commonsense and shared antagonism amongst many of its users.

Both the problem with, and the simple pertinence of, a social model is that the clue is in the name. Such models make distress, and how we handle it, everyone's responsibility all of the time; from the way we think about distress, through the way we organise society, to how we arrange care in our communities. Such models require us to examine the utility of some cherished ideas about the 'rights' of individuals over social responsibility. These examinations might be uncomfortable for psychotherapies that champion individual freedom above all else (Rose, 1996; Sanders and Tudor, 2001).

Within psychology, the possibilities of change might look scarce, but there are a few 'good news' stories. For example, the 'positive psychology' movement, instigated by Martin E. P. Seligman's Presidential Address to the American Psychological Association (APA) (Seligman, 1999) has had some success in transforming some ways of thinking. Seligman argued that, when it comes to understanding problems in living, a considerable amount of time and money has been spent over the years documenting the various ways in which people suffer psychologically, but that nowhere near the same effort has gone into understanding what makes life worth living, enjoyable, and meaningful. Seligman resolved to use his APA Presidency to initiate a shift in psychology's focus toward a more positive psychology. From these beginnings, the topic has become a magnet for research and a core topic in the mainstream psychology curriculum.

SOCIETY

Society's stock rises and falls with the zeitgeist, hitting rock-bottom on 31 October 1987 when Mrs Thatcher declared (when talking about 'disadvantaged' people to *Women's Own* magazine): 'They're casting their problem on society. And, you know, there is no such thing as society.'

Evidence shows that, whatever you call it, the way we structure our social and economic relations affects our biology and psychology, from the shamefully obvious (e.g. homeless people dying of hypothermia) to the insidious and unseen (e.g. UK children growing up in poverty are more likely to: have lower self-esteem; plan not to marry; believe that health is a matter of luck; play truant; expect to leave school at 16; have lower educational attainment; be unemployed as young adults; and experience psychological distress, compared to those who have never experienced poverty (Ermisch et al., 2001)).

A social model starts with the way we organise society. This is a complex network of material—economic, social, political—and psychological relations; the perception and understanding of which will be configured by our values. The history of social sciences is the struggle to unravel this tangle and it is not possible to do justice to this important issue in this brief chapter. However, a social model begins by looking at the social causes of distress (poverty, oppression, lack of opportunity, etc.) *and correcting them.* Easy to say, I know, and whether chicken or egg, the biologisation of experience and medicalisation of distress are obstacles to both our realisation of the nature of distress and the implementation of political solutions. So, with one foot in Utopia, assuming a programme of education and social reform is well under way, we can look at what a social model might be like in theory and practice.

A PERSON-CENTRED SOCIAL MODEL?

DEFICIENCY MODEL: DIAGNOSIS AND TREATMENT VS. POTENTIALITY MODEL:
UNDERSTANDING AND HELP

Models of distress work at four levels. The first concerns the *values* that underpin the approach. Once we have the values in sight they lead on to how we *understand* distress. Then we need a *method* for implementing the model and finally we have to be clear about how we *behave towards* distress. In the medical model, for example, we understand distress to be an illness. We collect data, apply calculations and then behave towards the illness by applying medical treatments to effect a cure. The values, methods, theory and behaviour should be harmonious—logically linked and with some level of face-validity. It wouldn't make much sense if we thought that distress was caused by a chemical imbalance, and that this would be corrected by exorcism.

A person-centred social model also has such domains: values which underpin the model, a way of thinking about the causes of distress, a method of discovery and a way of organising help. The remainder of this chapter will concentrate only partially on these elements, since its main aims are to stimulate interest in alternatives to the medical model of mental illness, to provide pointers to further reading and to suggest individual and collective action for counsellors and psychotherapists. It is not intended to be a balance sheet of the pros and cons of medical versus social models, or the differential effectiveness of social and psychological versus medical treatments.

Models of human experience (of which distress is only one element) have different ways of looking at the world.

- The *medical model* is reductionistic and locates the causes and resolutions of distress within the individual experiencing distress. The problem is in the person's 'pathology' which is 'cured' by medical interventions.
- Traditionally, the *person-centred approach* is holistic and growth-oriented, locating the causes of distress in social and interpersonal relationships and the resolution of distress within the individual's potential for positive growth. The problem is located in the way a person has grown to see the world which is 'grown through' by the actualising tendency when threat is removed.
- A *social model* is multi-disciplinary and holistic, locating the causes of distress in the social and material environment in which the individual lives (poverty; poor housing; lack of community services, employment, and opportunity; discrimination and structural oppression; violence, etc.), and their reaction to it (their biological[3] predisposition and psychology). The resolution of distress resides in changing the environment, helping the person come to terms with their biology and psychology or applying treatments (medical and psychological) where appropriate.

A social model with a person-centred methodology would be founded on principles of honesty, inclusiveness, equality of opportunity, holism, multidisciplinary enquiry and multidisciplinary management of helping opportunities. In addition to growing from person-centred organismic and psychological principles for therapeutic personality change, it would also enact PCA values in its organisation and implementation. It would put the distressed individual at the centre of a helping relationship dedicated to enhancing the agency of the individual and their involvement in controlling their own lives and, where appropriate, resolving their own distress.

In the PCA the healing process is characterised by organismic principles, i.e. that the organism—if given the right environmental conditions (importantly not limited to interpersonal conditions (Rogers 1959), but including social, economic and material conditions (Sanders, 2006b))—will actualise itself in the direction of growth, health and realisation of potential. This principle of life ensures that we must understand the many expressions of distress (terrifying and overwhelming as they are) as the reasonable organismic responses to an unreasonable and damaging world. This requires us to understand symptoms as self-protective coping strategies, however immediately unwelcome they are, rather like nausea and vomiting after ingesting a poison. In an inclusive social model, such

---

3. See footnote 1, p. 184.

understanding would be incorporated into a holistic strategy including improved opportunities for the person's material, social, physical and spiritual well-being.

Two other facets of person-centred psychology will impact on the nature of a social model. Although at a superficial level these simply restate familiar elements of theory, these notions must be integrated in a way which goes beyond the trivialisation which occurs in many trainings when these elements are reduced to skills. The first is that person-centred theory posits that there is one essential cause of distress—namely incongruence between the self-structure and experience—but that this is uniquely expressed by each organism. Only empathy and unconditional positive regard can address the uniqueness of the expression and resistance to change because of threat.

Second is the growing understanding of the dialogical nature of person-centred practice. Accounts can be found in the recent work of Godfrey Barrett-Lennard (2005); Dave Mearns (Mearns and Thorne, 2000; Mearns and Cooper, 2005); and Peter Schmid (1998, 2001a, b, c; 2002a), who has been foremost in elaborating person-centred dialogical therapy through the work of philosopher Emmanuel Levinas. One of the many consequences of a dialogical awareness is an appreciation of human beings as necessarily social and creative. The individual, understood as 'self-first', is no longer centre stage, since this approach emphasises the social context of therapy. It provides real philosophical foundations for a person-centred psycho-social practice in which 'putting the other first' becomes a viable philosophical position.

A person-centred social model is, therefore, multidisciplinary as it embraces the material, social, psychological, biological and spiritual aspects of being human. In particular then, a social model of distress:

- addresses the inner and outer worlds of individuals (including their macro-social, economic and material environments)
- embraces the social networks of distressed people
- promotes the need for empowerment and capacity building at a community level
- places equal value on the expertise of service users and carers
- develops and promotes a recovery model of mental distress—and a person-centred social model would include person-centred theory and practice
- resists simplification and reduction of the complexity of people's distress to a simple formula, mimicking the categorisation inherent in the medical model
- promotes *recovery*: 'The ability to live well in the presence or absence of ... whatever people choose to name their experience. Recovery happens when people with mental health problems take an active role in improving their lives, communities include them, and services enable the interaction.' (Wallcraft, in Tew, Beresford, Plumb, et al., 2002)
- adopts a positive psychological perspective because it is not simply concerned with the alleviation of distress and suffering, but also the promotion and facilitation of subjective and psychological well-being.

The implications of a social model are that all helpers wishing to work within a social model must:

- continue to develop an understanding of the nature of power, privilege and hierarchy in creating inequalities in, and exclusion from, opportunities to live fulfilling lives
- understand the psychological benefits of social capital
- work alongside service users and carers to promote their voices.

PSYCHO*SOCIAL* MODELS IN ACTION

I am now using the term 'psychosocial' to more accurately reflect its holistic inclusive nature. Some might argue that, to be precise, the model should be titled 'bio-psycho-social' but, for the purposes of this challenge, I am choosing to more properly reflect the true (i.e. marginal) influence of biological component as the evidence suggests[4] (for reviews see Pam, 1990; Cullberg, 2006, Read, Mosher and Bentall, 2004).

Persuading people that the current system is no longer fit for purpose, especially when it *appears* to serve the needs of a lot of people quite well, is not easy. The presentation of alternatives has its own pitfalls, in particular the tendency to be utopian and idealistic, since opportunities to evaluate alternatives in real life are few and far between. Readers will have to look beyond these difficulties and imagine what life might be like should a psychosocial model of distress be enacted. Notwithstanding these difficulties, there is a history of (sometimes rather isolated) alternatives to medicalised treatment, including recently, Ciompi (1997), Jenkinson (1999), Mosher and Hendrix (2004), and the continuing work of the Philadelphia Association (see <www.philadelphia-association.co.uk>) from which we can learn. Probably the best documented of these is Soteria House.

SOTERIA HOUSE

The closest to how the '"treatment" in a place of safety' end of a social model might operate in the real world can be found in the account of Soteria House. For a full history, description of principles and summary of research findings, readers are directed to *Soteria: Through Madness to Deliverance* (Mosher and Hendrix, 2004). In summary, Soteria House was established in 1971 as a residential psychiatric facility in a regular house in a multiethnic, working class community in San Jose, California, funded by the National Institute for Mental Health (NIMH), under the directorship of Loren Mosher. The elements of its operation relevant to this chapter are (see Mosher, 1999; Mosher and Hendrix, 2004):

Admissions policy
Patients selected to be at statistically high risk of developing a long-term condition, having to meet various criteria including:
- Diagnosed as *DSM-II* schizophrenia

---

4. See footnote 1, p. 184.

- In need of hospitalisation
- Exhibiting four of seven diagnostic symptoms of schizophrenia used by NIMH
- Single, aged 18–30
- Having no more than one previous hospitalisation.

On admission to hospital, patients were asked if they consented to taking part in a trial. They were then randomly allocated to Soteria House or local hospital acute psychiatric admissions ward for 'treatment as usual'. Admission to Soteria House was informal and individualised.

Staff
Non-professional staff; often with supplementary skills; cooking, carpentry, musicianship, massage. Selected after evaluation of how they related to 'psychotic' people. Instructed to not diagnose, interpret or behave like a psychotherapist. Trained to empathise, prevent unnecessary dependency, maintain patient autonomy and encourage patients to stay connected to their usual social networks and environments.

Relationship with community
Indistinguishable from other residences in the community. Interacts with and takes full part in the community.

Ethos
Home-like, safe. A recovery model (before such things were fashionable) built on *hope* and expectation of *recovery* (as opposed to expectation (indeed, almost *prescription*) of serious life-long illness with prognosis of chronic disability).

Treatments
'… the 24 hour-a-day application of interpersonal phenomenologic interventions by a non-professional staff, usually without neuroleptic drug treatment … the development of a non-intrusive, non-controlling but actively empathic relationship … "being with", "standing by attentively"' (Mosher, 1999: 37–8).

VIGNETTE

What follows is an imaginary situation in every sense of the word. Readers should not think that this is an example of how such a model *should* be or *should* work. It is just one way that a social model *might* operate in general and, in the case of this vignette, these particular, fictitious, lives. It is deliberately affected to illustrate how an ideal process might unfold. Some of the events may be shocking to psychologists, psychotherapists and counsellors used to working with an individualistic model in one-to-one therapy. To help with orientation, I suggest this quote from Pam Jenkinson, founder of the Wokingham Mind Crisis House:

There was, for instance, the consultant psychiatrist who tried to undermine our crisis house by criticising our lack of confidentiality ... Our role is not professional. We are *community* care and the community is not confidential. It is based on Mrs Smith meeting Mrs Jones in the High St and telling her that Mr Brown has had a fall and needs someone to get his shopping. It is dependent on knowing how everyone else is. (Jenkinson, 1999: 233. Original emphasis)

TERRY'S, TERRY'S FRIENDS', RELATIVES' AND NEIGHBOURS' STORY

Terry is a bright, seventeen year-old from a respectable working-class family. He has been a bit wayward, something of a character, from puberty but his escapades at school were becoming increasingly 'on the edge'. He is still the life and soul of the party, but his behaviour is becoming too strange, even for his closest friends. He drinks to excess and after a late night out with his friends he has been known to spend the night in bushes in strangers' gardens. He becomes more aggressive and climbs lamp-posts, shouting at traffic, passers-by and the world in general. He talks to himself and occasionally gets very agitated and his speech becomes jumbled. All of his behaviour causes concern to Joan, his mum, a single parent and committed church-goer, who, in desperation, asks for help from the priest.

Tom Smith, the parish priest, wasn't surprised when Joan came to see him. He, along with many others in the local community, had noticed that Terry's behaviour was becoming more and more disturbing. He had upset a few parishioners whom he had shouted at (mostly with his trademark impish, but on these occasions, inappropriate, smile) at the local shopping centre. Tom isn't an expert on psychological distress, but he recognises enough from Joan's description, and the rumours about Terry's behaviour, that Terry might need help. He has been here before and knows what to do—he asks Joan if he can visit their home when Terry is likely to be in.

The next day he visits and sits down with them both. He explains to Terry that his mum is worried and why. He tries to get Terry and Joan to talk about what is happening. He listens carefully to both of them and freely admits that he is not an expert. He is there as a priest and a friend. He suggests that they convene a 'circle of friends' for Terry. Terry knows what a circle of friends is for (they have lessons in citizenship at school), but he tells Tom and his mum that he is worried that it means he has done something wrong and will be punished. Tom reassures him and asks Terry who he thinks should be in the circle. The circle of friends should be tailored to the situation, so together they convene a small group comprising Terry; Jim, his friend from school; his form teacher; the family GP; Joan, Terry's mum; Tom, and the psychiatric social worker from the neighbourhood crisis house.

In the crisis house meeting room early the following week everyone gets to say something about their concerns, including Terry, who also has the opportunity of answering anything said about him. Sally, the social worker facilitates the meeting, since it was part of her training. She keeps the style of the meeting well within a caring atmosphere, largely because everyone really does care about Terry, even though a few of the people present are pissed-off with his behaviour. Terry is largely untouched by this, even when he hears from

Jim that friends at school are worried and frightened, thinking that he has gone over the top on a few occasions. After forthright exchanges, Terry, with his mum's support, agrees to the following suggestions:

• That someone from the family therapy team visits them at home to see if there is any help they can give Terry and his mum.

• That Terry sees a psychotherapist at the GP's surgery every week for an hour session.

• That the group meets again in a month, but before then, if things don't get any better at all, that Terry stays in the crisis house for a couple of weeks (if only to give Joan some respite from the worry that he might be getting into trouble).

• That Terry can go to the GP at any time to talk to someone about possible medications which might help. He will be told of the possible benefits and likely 'side' effects. Since Terry doesn't, at the moment, think there's much wrong from his point of view, he isn't impressed by this suggestion.

Three weeks later, however, the police bring Terry home on a Thursday afternoon because his behaviour outside the local chippy caused someone to dial 999. It wasn't exactly an emergency, and they responded with understanding once it was obvious that Terry was harmless. They were more concerned that he wasn't at school and, after some preliminary enquiries, they found out that he had a circle of friends. After a few frantic phone calls between Joan, Tom and Sally, Terry and Joan went down to the crisis house with Sally.

Terry stayed there for almost two weeks, during which time he got more and more agitated and anxious. A place was found in the residential facility only a couple of miles from his home where he could get 24-hour attention (the crisis house was for respite from life-stress rather than active care). The residential centre (similar to Soteria House) operated a therapeutic milieu where all the staff were trained to use contact reflections (Prouty, Van Werde and Pörtner, 2002) to make contact with residents and be sensitive to their needs. He saw a psychologist every day for a therapy session and could talk to support workers almost non-stop when the mood took him (there was a high staff–resident ratio). A peripatetic teacher employed by the local education authority for just such times, visited twice a week. His friends from school visited and were encouraged to keep him up to date with school work, even though Terry had difficulty in concentrating for very long. Everything was oriented towards his recovery and return to home and school.

Terry stayed for four months, during which time he experimented with taking some medication to ease his anxiety, but he didn't like it so stopped after a few days. He kept on seeing a psychotherapist at the GP's for about a year. Everyone thought his behaviour had calmed down and Terry himself became aware of the sort of things that triggered his agitated state and the thoughts which, to him, now seemed odd.

This is a simple story of shared responsibility and real connection between people— a community. Any one of the characters could have been in Terry's shoes. In fact, later that year, Sally's partner was killed in a car accident and she couldn't cope. Her family lived two hundred miles away so she had no immediate support. Her grief reaction was embraced by her chosen circle of friends and it took a couple of years support by a therapist at the GP practice for her to feel human again.

Do not be distracted by my choice of actors, since the priest who 'knows what to do' could just as easily be a youth worker, a shift manager at work, a neighbour, you or me. A social model is not built on professional power, but on all of us caring enough to know how everyone else is. This vignette is only utopian in the sense that it depends upon a tolerant society within which it can function properly. Save to say that the PCA principles of unconditional love and empathy lie at the heart of such social relations at all levels, this is not the place to debate such socio-political issues (see Rogers, 1961, 1978, 1980; Proctor, Cooper, Sanders and Malcolm, 2006). But our *actions* today and tomorrow in regard to the medicalisation of distress will determine whether the future for people like Terry (that means you and me) is a life on neuroleptic drugs and a trip to the ECT suite, or …

Readers wanting a glimpse of how to organise a humane approach to psychological distress could explore the down-to-earth ideas and practical approaches described by Loren Mosher and Lorenzo Burti (1994).

BUT WHAT ABOUT … ?

Difficult problems regarding behaviour have been airbrushed out of my vignette. Cynics may accuse me of using the same techniques as a drug company when it presents only the good results of its latest cure for the latest disorder. Violent or dangerous behaviour, class, crime, stigmatisation, individual freedom, safety and a host of other high profile issues impinge upon our understanding of distress and distressing people, none of which have been addressed in the vignette. But first we must separate the facts from the myths presented to us daily in the media—ever vigilant in their compulsion to associate 'mental illness' with crime, risk and danger—facts which often go 'missing in action' (Levin, 2005), when mental illness is in the news. Available space curtails further discussion here, so I suggest Thornicroft (2006) for further reading.

Then we have the problem of the structure of such a multidisciplinary system, how it will be funded, staffed and resourced. We can be sure that the stakeholders privileged by the current system may not give it their wholehearted support. But some will. There will be a need for honest expertise in pharmacology; key work and treatment plan management; various talking treatments; education and residential care. These people will have to learn to work in the genuine service of distressed people, their relatives and friends.

A further difficulty is the bourgeois picture of life, aspirations and opportunities I have painted. Poverty, lack of opportunity, lack of community services and other systemic deprivations are all absent. A reasonable criticism of the proposals implicit in the vignette (and the particular suggestion, borrowed from learning disability services, of a 'circle of friends') could be that this is fine for orderly, white middle-class families in safe neighbourhoods. However, it would have overcomplicated the vignette to locate it in a sink estate in north east Manchester, and been beyond my experience to set it in a minority ethnic community. I suggest that it is everyone's job to imagine, plan and organise how a social model might work *in detail* in different cultural settings; and that this job *has to be done* in order for the model to have any sense of being fit for the real world. How do you imagine it might work in practice where you live and work?

At risk of ad nauseam repetition, a social model must involve us all from the first moments of its inception to the discharge of its final responsibilities. There is nothing too awkward or unpleasant for inclusion and consideration. In fact it demands to be measured by how it embraces the extremes of human behaviour. And the 'it' of the model is 'us'. When supported by legislation, well staffed services and destigmatising education, we should all ask to be measured by how well we treat others in extreme distress.

WHAT TO DO NEXT

POSITIVE ACTION FOR PSYCHOLOGISTS, PSYCHOTHERAPISTS AND COUNSELLORS

Metaphor reassignment happens as a result of organised action, not by the unconnected acts of individuals. Women, gays and lesbians, and disabled people, organised, campaigned, lobbied, demonstrated, wrote articles and made change happen. That is the way the medical metaphor of distress will be changed. Psychotherapy and counselling in general, and the PCA in particular, have, however, let the idea of individual responsibility disconnect us from collective action. Our idea of community needs some adjustment. Unpopular though this message might be, the proof of the pudding can be found in the marginalisation of the PCA, whilst other better organised approaches seize the day.

I have been told that this last section is patronising. This may be a fair criticism. The suggestions in this last section are not 'instructions' to anyone other than myself. I do not assume that people are *not* already engaged in positive action in support of users of psychiatric services. However, at meetings of national and local groups dedicated to the humanisation of psychiatric services, psychotherapists and counsellors are conspicuous by their absence—outnumbered even by radical psychiatrists. So, looking first at the man in the mirror, here are some suggestions for positive action, involving coming out of the insular comfort of the PCA to say, 'I am against the medicalisation of distress and I'm person-centred. How can we work together on this?'

- Form special interest groups in professional bodies to campaign for constitutionally installed social, rather than medical, models for distress in counselling and psychotherapy
- Join with other like-minded helping professionals to campaign for a social model; social workers, psychologists, psychotherapists and critical psychiatrists
- Align with, and support, the service user movement; visit websites, subscribe to publications, go to meetings
- Challenge the medical model and psychodiagnosis at every possible turn
- Get involved with the user movement
- Be prepared to run groups, work with families and in communities and do other outreach work (and learn these skills where necessary)

- Actively work for the social inclusion of distressed people in our personal lives, our professional practice and the institutions in which we work
- Resist attempts to individualise and biologise problems—research psychosocial causes and psychosocial solutions with social science methodology, *not* pseudo-medical randomised controlled trials
- Revise theory and practice to accommodate social and other environmental factors
- Install this debate, with all of its awkwardness, at the centre of training in counselling, psychotherapy, psychology and psychiatry

There is no smart quote to conclude this chapter: it is now time to get involved; form our own opinions; debate with colleagues, friends and relatives; criticise this chapter; take action; join in ending the madness of the medical model.

REFERENCES

Barrett-Lennard, GT (2005) *Relationship at the Centre: Healing in a troubled world.* London: Whurr.

Bentall, RP (ed) (1990) *Reconstructing Schizophrenia.* London: Routledge.

Bentall, RP (2003) *Madness Explained: Psychosis and human nature.* London: Allen Lane/Penguin.

Boyle, M (1999) Diagnosis. In Newnes, G Holmes and C Dunn (eds) *This is Madness: A critical look at psychiatry and the future of mental health services* (pp. 75–90). Ross-on-Wye: PCCS Books.

Boyle, M (2002) *Schizophrenia: A scientific delusion.* London: Routledge.

Ciompi, L (1997) The Soteria concept: Theoretical bases and practices: 13-year experiences with a milieu-therapeutic approach to acute schizophrenia. *Psychiatrica et Neurologia Japanica, 9,* 634–50.

Coulter, J (1973) *Approaches to Insanity: A philosophical and sociological study.* New York: Wiley.

Cullberg, J (2006) *Psychoses: An integrative perspective.* London: Routledge.

Ermisch, J, Francesconi, M and Pevalin, DJ (2001) *Outcomes for Children of Poverty. DWP Research Report 158.* Leeds: Corporate Document Services, cited on <http://www.learningdisabilities. org.uk/page.cfm?pagecode=PIINCOPMEE>

Jenkinson, P (1999) The duty of community care: The Wokingham MIND crisis house. In Newnes, G Holmes and C Dunn (eds) *This is Madness: A critical look at psychiatry and the future of mental health services* (pp. 227–40). Ross-on-Wye: PCCS Books.

Harding, C, Brooks, G, Takamaru, A, Strauss, J and Breier, A (1987) The Vermont longitudinal study of persons with severe mental illness. *American Journal of Psychiatry, 144,* 718–35.

Harding, C and Zahnister, J (1994) Empirical correction of seven myths about schizophrenia with implication for treatment. *Acta Psychiatrica Scandinavia, 90 (Suppl. 384),* 140–6.

Levin, A (2005) When mental illness makes news, facts often missing in action. *Psychiatric News, 40,* 12, 18.

Maddux, JE, Snyder, CR and Lopez, SJ (2004) Toward a positive clinical psychology: Deconstructing the illness ideology and constructing an ideology of human strengths and potential. In PA Linley and S Joseph (eds) *Positive Psychology in Practice* (pp. 320–34). Hoboken, NJ: Wiley.

Madigan, S (1999) Inscription, description and deciphering chronic identities. In I Parker (ed) *Deconstructing Psychotherapy* (pp. 150–63). London: Sage.

Mearns, D (2006) Psychotherapy: The politics of liberation or collaboration? A career critically reviewed. In G Proctor, M Cooper, P Sanders and B Malcolm (eds) *Politicizing the Person-Centred Approach: An agenda for social change* (pp. 127–42). Ross-on-Wye: PCCS Books.

Mearns, D and Thorne, B (2000) *Person-Centred Therapy Today.* London: Sage.

Mearns, D and Cooper, M (2005) *Working at Relational Depth in Counselling and Psychotherapy.* London: Sage.

Mosher, LR (1999) Soteria and other alternatives to acute psychiatric hospitalization: A personal and professional view. *Changes, 17,* 35–51.

Mosher, LR and Burti, L (1994) *Community Mental Health: A practical guide.* London: Norton.

Mosher, L and Hendrix,V (2004) *Soteria: Through madness to deliverance.* Philadelphia: Xlibris.

Pam, A (1990) A critique of the scientific status of biological psychiatry. *Acta Psychiatrica Scandinavia Supplementum, 362,* 1–35.

Pilgrim, D and Rogers, A (2005) The troubled relationship between psychiatry and sociology. *International Journal of Social Psychiatry, 51,* 228–41.

Proctor, G, Cooper, M, Sanders, P and Malcolm, B (2006) *Politicizing the Person-Centred Approach: An agenda for social change.* Ross-on-Wye: PCCS Books.

Prouty, G, Van Werde, D and Pörtner, M (2002) *Pre-Therapy: Reaching contact-impaired clients.* Ross-on-Wye: PCCS Books.

Read, J and Haslam, N (2004) Public opinion: Bad things happen and can drive you crazy. In J Read, LR Mosher and RP Bentall, *Models of Madness: Psychological, social and biological approaches to schizophrenia,* (pp. 133–46). Hove: Brunner-Routledge.

Read, J, Mosher, L and Bentall, RP (2004) *Models of Madness: Psychological, social and biological approaches to schizophrenia.* Hove: Brunner-Routledge.

Rogers, CR (1959) A theory of therapy, personality and interpersonal relationships as developed in the client-centered framework. In S Koch (ed) *Psychology: The Study of a Science, Vol. 3.* (pp. 184–256). New York: McGraw-Hill.

Rogers, CR (1961) *On Becoming a Person.* Boston: Houghton Mifflin.

Rogers, CR (1978) *Carl Rogers on Personal Power.* London: Constable.

Rogers, CR (1980) *A Way of Being.* Boston: Houghton Mifflin.

Rose, N (1996) *Inventing Our Selves: Psychology, power and personhood.* Cambridge: Cambridge University Press.

Sanders, P (2005) Principled and strategic opposition to the medicalisation of distress and all of its apparatus. In S Joseph and R Worsley (eds) *Person-Centred Psychopathology: A positive psychology of mental health,* (pp. 21–42). Ross-on-Wye: PCCS Books.

Sanders, P (2006a) The spectacular self: Alienation as the lifestyle choice of the free world, endorsed by psychotherapists. In G Proctor, M Cooper, P Sanders and B Malcolm (eds) *Politicizing the Person-Centred Approach: An agenda for social change,* (pp. 95–114). Ross-on-Wye: PCCS Books.

Sanders, P (2006b) Why person-centred therapists must reject the medicalisation of distress. *Self and Society 34,* 32–39.

Sanders, P (2007) Schizophrenia is not an illness: A response to van Blarikom. *Person-Centered and Experiential Psychotherapies 6,* 112–28.

Sanders, P and Tudor, K (2001) This is therapy: A person-centred critique of the contemporary psychiatric system. In C Newnes, G Holmes and C Dunn (eds) *This is Madness Too: Critical perspectives on mental health services* (pp. 147–60). Ross-on-Wye: PCCS Books.

Sargent, W (1966) Recovery rates from schizophrenia prior to the introduction of neuroleptic medication. Paper delivered to the Royal College of Psychiatrists.

Schmid, PF (1998) 'Face to face'—the art of encounter. In B Thorne and E Lambers (eds) *Person-Centred Therapy: A European perspective* (pp. 74–90). London: Sage.

Schmid, PF (2001a) Authenticity: The person as his or her own author. Dialogical and ethical perspectives on therapy as an encounter relationship. And beyond. In G Wyatt (ed) *Rogers' Therapeutic Conditions: Evolution, theory and practice. Vol. 1: Congruence,* (pp. 217–32). Ross-on-Wye: PCCS Books.

Schmid, PF (2001b) Comprehension: The art of not-knowing. Dialogical and ethical perspectives on empathy as dialogue in personal and person-centred relationships. In S Haugh and T Merry (eds) *Rogers' Therapeutic Conditions: Evolution, theory and practice. Vol. 2: Empathy* (pp. 53–71). Ross-on-Wye: PCCS Books.

Schmid, PF (2001c) Acknowledgement: The art of responding. Dialogical and ethical perspectives on the challenge of unconditional personal relationships in therapy and beyond. In J Bozarth and P Wilkins (eds) *Rogers' Therapeutic Conditions: Evolution, theory and practice. Vol. 3: Unconditional Positive Regard* (pp. 49–64). Ross-on-Wye: PCCS Books.

Schmid, PF (2002a) Presence: Im-media-te co-experiencing and co-responding. Phenomeno-logical, dialogical and ethical perspectives on contact and perception in person-centred therapy and beyond. In G Wyatt and P Sanders (eds) *Rogers' Therapeutic Conditions: Evolution, theory and practice. Vol. 4: Contact and Perception* (pp. 182–203). Ross-on-Wye: PCCS Books.

Seligman, MEP (1999) The president's address. *American Psychologist, 54,* 559–62.

Seligman, MEP (2003) *Authentic Happiness: Using the new positive psychology to realize your potential for lasting fulfilment.* New York: Free Press.

Tew, J, Beresford, P, Plumb, S, Ferns, P, Wallcraft, J, Williams, J and Carr, S (2002) *Start Making Sense … Developing social models to understand and work with mental distress.* Published for the Social Perspectives Network by TOPSS. Downloaded from <http://www.spn.org.uk/fileadmin/SPN_uploads/Documents/Papers/SPN_Papers/spn_paper_3.pdf>.

Thornicroft, G (2006) *Shunned: Discrimination against people with mental illness.* Oxford: Oxford University Press.

UNICEF (2007) *Report Card 7, Child Poverty in Perspective: An overview of child well-being in rich countries.* Downloaded from <http://www.unicef-icdc.org/presscentre/presskit/reportcard7/rc7_eng.pdf>.

Wing, JK (1978) *Reasoning About Madness.* Oxford: Oxford University Press.

CHAPTER 17

OUTCOME MEASUREMENT IN PERSON-CENTRED PRACTICE

Thomas G. Patterson and Stephen Joseph

INTRODUCTION

Over recent years we have witnessed a growing climate of pressure on counsellors, psychologists and psychotherapists to produce evidence of the effectiveness of their therapeutic practice. This demand, which has become ubiquitous in the therapeutic professions, presents particular difficulties for person-centred practitioners who understand that *what works* in counselling and psychotherapy principally concerns relationship variables and the activation of a growth-oriented process in the client, rather than specific techniques aimed at symptom alleviation as an end goal of therapy. In this chapter, we aim to address some of the main challenges facing person-centred practitioners by proposing that evaluating therapeutic change does not have to undermine the principles of the person-centred approach and should not be limited to the measurement of symptom reduction as the only valid indicator of therapeutic effectiveness. We argue that through adopting a creative and proactive attitude to outcome evaluation, person-centred practitioners could identify and introduce theoretically and ethically congruent ways of demonstrating the effectiveness of client-centred therapy and counselling, that also answer demands from healthcare providers for outcome evaluation.

EVALUATING THERAPEUTIC EFFECTIVENESS

An increasing emphasis on the provision of psychological therapies that have a clear evidence base has meant that funding decisions for therapy provision are now strongly influenced by research reviews and clinical practice guidelines. Obviously, reviews of the effectiveness of different types of psychotherapy will reflect findings for psychological therapies where outcomes have been extensively researched and, until now, these have tended to be the more structured and symptom-focussed approaches such as cognitive-behavioural therapy. Not surprisingly, it has been argued that all the humanistic therapies, with their focus on the whole person and not just specific symptoms, will be *empirically violated* by the emphasis of research on treatments targeted for specific disorders, an approach to outcome evaluation that is inherently biased in favour of more medicalised approaches to therapy (see Bohart, O'Hara and Leitner, 1998).

The use of such outcome studies as a guide to therapeutic effectiveness is a source of debate among practitioners. While there is a certain amount of evidence to support the effectiveness of condition-specific interventions (see Roth and Fonagy, 1996), there is also much evidence to suggest that the empirical support for condition-specific treatments remains unproven (see for example, King, 1998; Bozarth, 2002; Hubble and Miller, 2004). Furthermore, at a more fundamental level, there is increasing evidence to suggest that even the use of psychiatric diagnostic categories around which condition-specific interventions are organised is itself intrinsically flawed (see Bentall, 2003). In addition, it is becoming increasingly clear that the various psychotherapies are all effective to approximately the same degree. This general equivalence of the different approaches to psychotherapy is evidenced by findings from a recent examination of seventeen meta-analyses of treatment comparisons showing that results indicating differences in therapeutic effectiveness between the various forms of psychotherapy were so small as to be statistically meaningless (Luborsky, Rosenthal, Diguer, Andrusyna, Berman, Levitt *et al.*, 2002). These findings are consistent with the results of a similar review carried out twenty-seven years earlier (Luborsky, Singer and Luborsky, 1975).

THE PERSON-CENTRED VIEW OF THERAPEUTIC CHANGE

Client-centred therapy, in line with its person-centred theoretical base, proposes that the *client* and the *relationship* are the active ingredients of change in counselling and psychotherapy (Rogers, 1951, 1957a, 1959; Bozarth, 1998). A failure to acknowledge the contribution of therapeutic relationship factors to therapy outcomes appears to go hand in hand with the current focus of outcome research on disorder-specific treatments (Bohart *et al.*, 1998; Bozarth, 2002; Cornelius-White, 2002). This failure is surprising given consistent findings from reviews of outcome research indicating that approximately thirty per cent of the variance in outcome across therapies is accounted for by client-therapist relationship variables compared to fifteen per cent accounted for by specific techniques (with forty per cent of variance explained by extra-therapeutic or client factors) (Lambert, 1992; Lambert and Barley, 2001; Lambert, Shapiro and Bergin, 1986). These findings are consistent with Patterson's earlier report that empathy, warmth and genuineness account for between twenty-five and forty per cent of outcome variance (Patterson, 1984), and they support person-centred theory's assertion that the therapeutic relationship and the client's resources are the critical variables in effective therapy (Rogers, 1951, 1957a, 1959). More recently, the American Psychological Association Division 29 Task Force on Empirically Supported Therapy Relationships found that all of the general relationship variables it reviewed, including the person-centred variables of empathy, positive regard, and congruence-genuineness, were either demonstrably effective or promising, and probably effective in terms of achieving successful therapeutic outcome (Ackerman, Benjamin, Beutler, Gelso, Goldfried, Hill et al., 2001; Cornelius-White, 2002).

While research into the process of therapeutic change has a considerable history within the person-centred tradition (see Barrett-Lennard, 1998; Bozarth, Zimring and

Tausch, 2002), the symptom-reduction focus of more contemporary outcome studies in psychotherapy has predominantly relied on medical-like indicators of therapeutic effectiveness as defined by psychiatric terminology. Consequently, recent studies of the therapeutic effectiveness of client-centred therapy have not concerned themselves with theoretically congruent indicators of change, such as testing for the development of unconditional positive self-regard, but have instead tended to evaluate the degree of symptom alleviation achieved. Even given this limitation, client-centred therapy fares extremely well in such research (see Elliott, 1996; Friedli, King, Lloyd and Horder, 1997; King, Sibbald, Ward, Bower, Lloyd, Gabbay and Byford, 2000, for example).

However, person-centred theory offers an alternative positive psychological paradigm to the medical model in which distress and dysfunction are not viewed as clinically separate disorders, but as expressions of thwarted potential as the organism self-actualises incongruently in respect of its actualising tendency. In this way it provides a holistic framework for understanding both the negative and the positive aspects of human experience (see Joseph and Worsley, 2005a). Rather than being difficult to evaluate, it is perhaps more accurate to say that an approach grounded in a humanistic theory and one which explicitly opposes the medicalisation of psychological distress ought not to be evaluated in a manner determined by an approach that is grounded in biomedical theory. That said, the pressure remains for client-centred counsellors and therapists to provide evidence of the effectiveness of their approach if their invaluable contribution to promoting psychological well-being is not to go overlooked by healthcare funders and providers. We propose that the development and use of self-report measurement scales designed to assess process-outcome variables beyond the symptom-reduction paradigm could play a role in the resolution of this difficult dilemma.

DECIDING WHAT TO MEASURE

An essential question for any practitioner to consider is what exactly he or she is being asked to measure when outcome evaluation is proposed. Client-centred counsellors and therapists take a radically different view of therapeutic change than practitioners from many other approaches in that they do not consider symptom reduction to be the central goal of therapy. They aim instead to set in motion a process of change in a growth-oriented direction. According to this conceptualisation, outcome is seen as a process instead of a fixed single end-point. Thus, while a measure of presence or absence of anxiety symptoms might be appropriate for an intervention that aims to reduce anxiety, it will not serve the same purpose within a client-centred intervention where process changes and outcomes are intertwined and where a successful outcome is one in which the process of change has begun, is ongoing and will continue into the future beyond symptom reduction. In this way, client-centred therapy is not just concerned with the alleviation of symptoms but is also concerned with the facilitation of positive growth and personal development that underpins people's strivings to become more fully functional. As Bozarth (1998) wrote:

> The individual's return to unconditional positive self-regard is the crux of psychological growth in the theory. It is the factor that reunifies the self with the actualising tendency. (Bozarth, 1998: 84)

Rogers (1959) identified the key indicators of successful therapy to be increased congruence, increased openness to experience, and reduced defensiveness. Other positive indicators of change include an increase in unconditional positive self-regard, an increase in autonomy and self-trusting, and a reduction in conditions of worth. These are all constructs that can be operationalised and measured. As Rogers (1959) points out, the person-centred theory of therapy is an *if–then* theory wherein, given the presence of necessary and sufficient social-environmental conditions within the context of the therapeutic relationship, certain measurable process-changes and outcomes will occur. This suggests that there are few obstacles to prevent the development of theoretically grounded outcome measures that evaluate therapeutic change and effectiveness in terms of the process-outcomes predicted by the person-centred theory of therapy.

In our view, appropriate outcome measures should seek to evaluate changes in such variables as unconditional positive self-regard, conditions of worth, openness to experience (reduced defensiveness), existential living (living in the 'here and now'), autonomy (self-determination), psychological growth or well-being and trust in self. Such measures could provide a way of evaluating the effectiveness of client-centred therapy without undermining the theoretical basis of the approach. All these indicators of therapeutic growth are to some degree attitudinal and as such are amenable to measurement. Even though self-report scales only provide a cross-sectional snapshot of the person's attitudinal position (such as degree of openness to experience) at a fixed point in time, repeating this measurement at various points throughout therapy can provide both client and practitioner with valuable information about the process of change in the client (e.g. at pre-intervention, during intervention, and post-intervention). In this way, such measures can act as an additional source of feedback for practitioners and their clients about the client's progress as well as addressing external demands to systematically monitor and evaluate therapeutic practice.

One final consideration relates to previously highlighted concerns about the question of empirical violation. More recently, and in particular over the last decade, there has been an increasing move across all contexts of healthcare provision to specifically evaluate therapy outcomes. For this reason it is now becoming more important that rating scales are developed that can measure the process of growth-oriented change in client-centred therapy. Otherwise, the person-centred approach risks becoming increasingly marginalised due to the biased approach to outcome evaluation that is grounded in the currently dominant biomedical paradigm. As previously mentioned, Bohart and colleagues point to the risk that person-centred theory may be empirically violated by moves to establish support for psychotherapies that are based on a medicalised, symptom-reduction paradigm (Bohart et al.,1998). This is consistent with Carl Rogers' own criticisms of logical positivism in his later career (see Rogers, 1985). Logical positivism asserts that there is a neutral language of scientific observation which allows for objective comparison of different scientific theories. Reliance on symptom-reduction as the core indicator of therapeutic effectiveness carries with it the assumption that symptom-reduction is a neutral concept that is shared by all the various therapeutic approaches. This assumption of neutral objectivity is clearly beneficial to proponents of the medical model paradigm, but it has long since been shown to be erroneous (see Popper, 1959/1980). Furthermore, Kuhn (1962/1996) has shown that the criterion for choice between competing theories is never logical as there is no neutral language of observation or shared basic vocabulary between theories. Consequently, terms such as *proof* and *truth* cannot be applied in inter-theoretical contexts. A more holistic approach, such as the person-centred one, involves a very particular set of assumptions which, in turn, demand a particular set of social and therapeutic responses.

In this respect we agree with Pfaffenberger (2006) who asserts that there is a need to highlight the limitations of the positivistic paradigm, arguing that the light of social-constructivist informed critical theory must be brought to bear on the findings of therapeutic outcome research. However, we also believe that a complete rejection of quantitative research methodologies, such as the use of rating scales in outcome research, is tantamount to throwing out the baby (quantitative methodologies) with the bathwater (logical positivism). We argue that making use of theoretically congruent self-report measurement scales provides one way of collecting data about therapeutic change that can complement qualitative approaches to data collection and will also contribute to the development of a discourse on outcome evaluation that is rooted in person-centred theory, that uses the language and concepts of the theory, and that will help to redress the current one-sidedness in this area of research.

OUTCOME MEASUREMENT SCALES

DEVELOPMENT OF OUTCOME EVALUATION IN CLIENT-CENTRED THERAPY

A number of rating scales have been developed over the years to measure therapeutic change in accordance with the predictions of person-centred personality theory (see Barrett-Lennard, 1998, for comprehensive overview of this research). The earliest studies of the process of therapeutic change were carried out in the 1940s and relied on the evaluation of transcripts of therapist–client interviews using a content analytic approach (e.g. Snyder, 1945). A shift to studying outcome using data external to the interview process emerged in the late 1940s and early 1950s with the use of projective tests pre- and post-therapy (e.g. Carr, 1949). The use of client self-rating methods to investigate the change process was a feature of person-centred research in the early 1950s, with both the introduction of the Q-sort method for ranking a series of self-descriptive statements (e.g. Butler and Haigh, 1954) and the use of self-report attitudinal scales such as the Self-Other Scale (Gordon and Cartwright , 1954). Although a considerable evidence base for client-centred therapy was developed by person-centred researchers throughout the 1950s and 1960s (see Barrett-Lennard, 1998), Carl Rogers' own move away from the academic world of the university was followed by a decline in the level of research into client-centred therapy. Nonetheless, there have been a few attempts over the years to develop self-report rating scales based on person-centred theory that can provide quantitative information about the process of change in client-centred therapy (see for example, Cartwright and Mori,1988; Betz, Wohgelmuth, Serling, Harshbarger and Klein, 1995). A number of self-report scales have also been developed to measure the self-actualisation process based on broader humanistic conceptualizations of self-actualisation that reflect the theoretical work of both Abraham Maslow and Carl Rogers (see, for example, Shostrom, 1966a; Sorochan, 1976; Lefrancois, Leclerc, Dube, Herbert, and Gaulin, 1997).

The most widely used of the aforementioned measures is the Personal Orientation Inventory (POI) (Shostrom, 1966a), a one hundred and fifty-item scale that is composed of the two subscales of *time competence* and *inner directedness*. Time competence is a measure of ability to live in the 'here and now' (Shostrom, 1966a). A person high in this factor will, characteristically, be less anxious, have less feelings of guilt, have few regrets about the past, and will have goals that are meaningfully tied to current goal pursuits (Shostrom, 1966a). The second subscale of inner directedness provides a measure that reflects a reactivity orientation that is directed toward the self so that the person acts in a manner that is relatively autonomous from the influence of others (Shostrom, 1966b). A number of research studies have confirmed the validity of the POI (e.g. Shostrom and Knapp, 1967; Fox, Knapp and Michael, 1968).

Although the POI is well validated and could potentially be applied to the context of outcome evaluation, one limitation of the measure is that, due to the large number of scale items, it takes approximately thirty-five to forty-five minutes to complete and would therefore be relatively burdensome for clients in terms of time demands. This fact may discourage many practitioners from making use of it. Carver (1997) has argued that the development of shorter, less time-consuming measures is one way of reducing participant response burden in terms of time and effort, and of increasing the likelihood that such measures will be used for research in applied settings. We agree that brief scales are a bonus for both clients and practitioners and, in light of this consideration, the present overview of outcome measures aims to focus on briefer self-report measures that are less time-consuming than the POI.

BRIEF MEASUREMENT SCALES FOR OUTCOME EVALUATION

As previously mentioned, the aim of this chapter is to provide an overview of outcome measures that could be used by person-centred practitioners to evaluate their therapeutic practice. We will begin by describing a new measure of unconditional positive self-regard recently developed by ourselves (Patterson and Joseph, 2006). Following this, we will provide an overview of a number of existing self-report measures that, while not developed specifically as person-centred outcome measures, do nonetheless appear to fit well with the need of client-centred counsellors and therapists for outcome measures that are consistent with the theoretical assumptions of the person-centred approach.

MEASURING UNCONDITIONAL POSITIVE SELF-REGARD

A key therapeutic goal of client-centred therapy is to achieve a loosening of the client's rigid internalised rules and values in order to allow the client freedom to grow and develop. This is facilitated by the creation of necessary and sufficient relationship conditions within the therapeutic encounter (Rogers, 1957a). Person-centred theory argues that it is through establishing and maintaining these relationship conditions that the client is enabled to achieve positive therapeutic change, evidenced by an increase in the individual's unconditional positive self-regard and a decrease in conditions of worth (Rogers, 1959).

The Unconditional Positive Self-Regard Scale
The Unconditional Positive Self-Regard Scale (UPSRS) (Patterson and Joseph, 2006) is based on Rogers' (1959) formal definition of unconditional positive self-regard (UPSR):

> When the individual perceives himself in such a way that no self-experience can be discriminated as more or less worthy of positive regard than any other, then he is experiencing unconditional positive self-regard. (Rogers, 1959: 209)

According to this definition, there are two distinguishable facets of UPSR. The first element refers to the expression or withholding of positive regard towards oneself, or positive self-regard. Whether or not positive self-regard is expressed is conditional upon the individual's perception of his or her self-experiences as differentially worthy of positive regard, in turn determined by internalised conditions of worth. This conditionality, or conditional–unconditional continuum, appears to be the second element of the construct of UPSR as defined. It follows then that items designed to measure UPSR should refer to both of these facets of the construct—*positive self-regard* and *conditionality* of positive self-regard. A similar operational distinction was adopted by Barrett-Lennard (1962, 1986) when developing a measure of the conceptually related construct of unconditional positive regard, and for this reason the generation of scale items for the UPSRS was based on Barrett-Lennard's earlier work (see Patterson and Joseph, 2006.)

The scale consists of twelve items—six that measure the person's level of positive self-regard (self-regard subscale) and six that measure level of unconditional self-regard (conditionality subscale), with interviewees' responses to the items being scored on a five-point Likert-type scale ranging from 'strongly agree' to 'strongly disagree'. After taking reverse scored items into account, a total score for each subscale is calculated by summing the subscale item scores. Extensive psychometric work carried out in the development of the UPSRS showed that the scale has a two-factor structure, acceptable levels of internal consistency reliability (Cronbach's alpha = .88 for the Self-Regard subscale and .79 for the Conditionality subscale), good construct validity and good convergent and discriminant validity in relation to other measures (see Patterson and Joseph, 2006). A full copy of the UPSRS with instructions for administering and scoring is provided at the end of this chapter (see Appendix). The UPSRS provides a quick and easy-to-administer measure of therapeutic outcome in a format that is minimally burdensome to potential clients and is therefore appropriate for use in applied settings. Although there remains a need for further validation studies, the scale offers person-centred practitioners a useful way of evaluating client change in counselling or psychotherapy.

In the following sections, we briefly review some other measures which are grounded in, or consistent with, person-centred theory. It is not a systematic review of available measures but serves as an illustration of the different resources that are available, drawn from the literatures on social psychology and positive psychology.

MEASURING CONDITIONS OF WORTH

'Conditions of worth' refer to the internalised rules and values upon which the individual's self-regard has become contingent (Rogers, 1959). Until recently, there has been no way of measuring Rogerian conditions of worth. However, a self-report scale recently developed by researchers concerned with understanding self-esteem appears to hold particular relevance for person-centred practitioners interested in studying changes in conditions of worth.

The Contingencies of Self-Worth Scale

Contingencies of self-worth represent a construct that is conceptually very similar to person-centred conditions of worth. The Contingencies of Self-Worth Scale (CSWS) (Crocker, Luhtanen, Cooper, and Bouvrette, 2003) was designed to measure the degree to which a person's level of self-esteem is tied to subjectively valued domains of interpersonal and intrapsychic goals, standards or expectations. As such, the individual's feelings of self-worth, or self-esteem, are considered to be contingent upon perceived success or failure in those particular domains in which self-esteem is invested. Consequently, behavioural and emotional self-regulation is governed by attempts to achieve success and avoid failure in the valued domains, resulting in defensive responses when contingent domains are threatened (Crocker and Wolfe, 2001; Crocker, Luhtanen, Cooper, and Bouvrette, 2003). According to this definition, contingencies of self-worth appear to be conceptually very similar, if not identical, to conditions of worth: 'When any expression of self is avoided or sought solely because of its effect on self-regard, the person is said to have acquired a *condition of worth*.' (Barrett-Lennard,1998: 77).

The CSWS is a thirty-five-item scale designed to assess seven sources of self-worth (others' approval, appearance, competition, academic competence, family support, virtue, God's love). Example items include: 'When my family members are proud of me, my sense of self-worth increases', or, 'My self-worth is influenced by how well I do on competitive tasks'. Responses are given on a seven-point Likert-type scale and are then summed for each subscale. The seven subscales all have high internal consistency (Cronbach's alpha values range from .82 to .96), and a three month test-retest reliability ranging from .68 to .92 (Crocker et al., 2003).

MEASURING AUTONOMY

Rogers (1957b) coined the term *fully functioning person* to describe a state of more optimal psychological functioning that occurs when self-actualisation and the actualising tendency are concordant. The term captures the contrast between process and stasis, describing the individual who is a continually changing person-in-process (Rogers, 1959). The development of increasing autonomy is characteristic of the more fully functioning person. Person-centred theory's conceptualisation of organismically congruent self-actualisation is described as involving '... the development toward autonomy and away from heteronomy, or control by external forces' (Rogers,1959:196). Autonomy in person-centred theory is synonymous with internal freedom—the psychological freedom to move in any direction—and it develops in line with the individual's increasing organismic valuing.

Self-Determination Scale

The Self-Determination Scale (SDS) (Sheldon and Deci, 1996) was designed to assess individual differences in the extent to which people tend to function in a more autonomous or self-determined way. Self-Determination is synonymous with more autonomous functioning, posited by Rogers (1959) as one of the key goals of client-centred therapy, and self-determination theory holds similar meta-theoretical assumptions to person-centred theory (see Patterson and Joseph, 2007). The SDS has been shown to have two factors: *self-contact* or awareness of oneself (being more aware of one's feelings and sense of self); and *choicefulness* or perceived choice (feeling a sense of choice with respect to one's behaviour) (Sheldon, Ryan, and Reis, 1996). The ten-item scale is composed of two five-item subscales. For each item, participants indicate which of two statements feels most true for them; e.g. (a) 'My emotions sometimes seem alien to me' versus (b) 'My emotions always seem to belong to me' (a self-contact item) or a) 'I sometimes feel that it's not really me choosing the things I do' versus (b) 'I always feel like I choose the things I do' (a choicefulness item). Participants respond to each item by scoring from one to nine on a Likert-type scale and, after recoding reversed items, responses are then added together. The subscales can either be used separately or combined into an overall SDS score. The SDS has been psychometrically evaluated and shown to have good internal consistency, adequate test-retest reliability, and to be a strong predictor of a wide variety of psychological health outcomes, including self-actualisation, empathy and life satisfaction (Sheldon and Deci, 1996). It has also been used in a number of published research studies (Sheldon, 1995; Sheldon, Ryan, and Reis, 1996; Elliot and McGregor, 2001).

MEASURING EXISTENTIAL LIVING

Rogers' (1961) observed that one of the main process-changes to occur in more fully functioning individuals is a movement towards more *existential living* or living in the *here and now*:

> A second characteristic of the process which for me is the good life, is that it involves an increasing tendency to live fully in each moment. Such living in the moment means an absence of rigidity, of tight organization of the imposition of structure on experience. It means instead a maximum of adaptability, a discovery of structure in experience, a flowing, changing organization of self and personality ... It involves discovering the structure of experience *in* the process of living the experience. To open one's spirit to what is going on *now*, and to discover in that present process whatever structure it appears to have—this to me is one of the qualities of the good life, the mature life, as I see clients approach it. (1961: 188–189)

The construct of Mindfulness refers to the development of the ability to pay deliberate attention to our experience in the present moment, non-judgementally. It has been described as '... an open or receptive awareness of and attention to what is taking place in the present moment' (Brown and Ryan, 2004: 116). Our opinion is that mindfulness is analogous to the process-outcome of existential living that Rogers observed to be characteristic of more fully functioning clients.

Mindfulness Attention Awareness Scale

The Mindfulness Attention Awareness Scale (MAAS) (Brown and Ryan, 2003) operationalises the construct of mindfulness in dispositional terms, and we believe it could provide a useful and theoretically congruent measure of more positive, optimal functioning in clients. It is a fifteen-item self-report instrument with a single factor structure. For each item, participants are asked to indicate how frequently or infrequently they have various experiences. Responses are on a Likert-type scale going from one (almost always) to six (almost never). An overall scale score is obtained by calculating the mean score for the fifteen items. Higher scores reflect higher levels of dispositional mindfulness. Examples of items include: 'I could be experiencing some emotion and not be conscious of it until some time later', 'I find it difficult to stay focused on what's happening in the present', and 'I tend not to notice feelings of physical tension or discomfort until they really grab my attention'. The scale has been validated in populations of college students, working adults and cancer patients, showing reasonable convergent and discriminant validity, strong internal consistency and adequate test-retest reliability (Brown and Ryan, 2003).

GROWTH-ORIENTED MEASUREMENT OF CHANGES IN PSYCHOPATHOLOGY

Our view of person-centred theory is that it offers a holistic paradigm, integrative of both negative and positive aspects of human experience. While we argue for non-medicalised outcome measures, we do not accept criticisms that the person-centred approach is not relevant to more severe psychopathology. Rather, we take the view that client-centred therapists work holistically with psychopathology, aiming to facilitate psychological well-being through engaging with the constructive, growth-oriented actualising tendency and the client's organismic valuing process. Inasmuch as absence of medicalised symptoms is correlated with increased well-being, symptom reduction is likely to occur as part of the process of client-centred therapy, but it is neither the goal of therapy nor is it considered an end-point in the client's process of change. A comprehensive exploration of the application of the person-centred approach to psychopathology can be found elsewhere (see Joseph and Worsley, 2005a). Here we will restrict ourselves to a consideration of two outcome measures that can be used to evaluate changes in psychopathology in a manner that focuses on growth-oriented change.

Short Depression–Happiness Scale

The Short Depression–Happiness Scale (SDHS) (Joseph, Linley, Harwood, Lewis and McCollam, 2004) differs from traditional self-report measures of depression in that, as well as giving an indication of the degree of alleviation of depression, it also provides a measure of the extent to which the client is moving towards more happy and satisfied living. This is consistent with the focus on the facilitation of positive growth and development beyond symptom-reduction that is characteristic of client-centred therapy. The SDHS is a six-item self-report questionnaire that provides a measure of the continuum of depression-happiness. The scale does not define depression in terms of DSM diagnostic categories but, instead, refers to a general reduced affect and loss of vitality. Three of the questionnaire items ask about positive thoughts, feelings and bodily experiences (e.g. I felt pleased with the way I am), while the other three items ask about negative thoughts, feelings and bodily experiences (I felt dissatisfied with my life). Respondents are asked to think about how they have felt in the past seven days and to rate the frequency of each item on a four-point scale: never (0), rarely (1), sometimes (2) and often (3). Items concerning negative thoughts, feelings and bodily experiences are reverse scored so that when all six items are summed, respondents can potentially score between nought and eighteen, with higher scores indicating greater frequency of positive thoughts and feelings and lower frequency of negative thoughts and feelings. The average score is around twelve. The scale has been extensively validated through psychometric evaluation to confirm that it has a single-factor structure, acceptable levels of internal consistency reliability, and convergent validity with other measures (see Joseph and Lewis, 1998; Joseph et al., 2004).

Growth following traumatic stress: Changes in Outlook Questionnaire

The topic of traumatic stress has been conceptualised from the person-centred approach, leading to the new understanding that the natural end point of emotional processing following trauma is growth (Joseph, 2003, 2004, 2005; Joseph and Linley, 2005). A variety of measures have been developed to assess personal growth and positive change through adversity. The first such measure to be developed was the Changes in Outlook Questionnaire (CiOQ) originally developed by Joseph, Williams and Yule (1993). The CiOQ provides a self-report assessment of the extent to which a person has experienced both positive changes and negative changes following adversity and trauma. The CiOQ consists of twenty-six items; eleven assess positive changes and fifteen assess negative changes. The eleven positive items are summed to give a total score ranging from eleven to sixty-six. The fifteen negative items are summed to give a total score ranging from fifteen to ninety. The CiOQ has been extensively psychometrically validated and promises to be useful tool when working with clients who have experienced trauma and adversity (Joseph et al., 2005). For practitioners who may need brief and quick-to-administer measures, a short version of the CiOQ is also available (Joseph, Linley, Shevlin, Goodfellow and Butler, 2006).

CONCLUSION

The person-centred view is that psychotherapy, in its essence, is a personal transaction, a growth-facilitating relationship that takes place within a clearly defined and boundaried context and that approaches the client holistically, as a person rather than a set of medicalised symptoms or a diagnostic category. A non-medicalised approach to outcome measurement therefore flows logically from the theoretical stance of client-centred therapy, where establishing the *necessary and sufficient relationship conditions,* and an emphasis on working within the client's *frame of reference,* are given primacy (Rogers, 1957a, 1959). In providing an introduction to a number of existing measurement scales that appear to lend themselves well to use by client-centred counsellors and therapists, it has been argued that proactive efforts by person-centred practitioners to make use of theoretically congruent and growth-oriented measures of therapeutic change could facilitate the evaluation of client-centred therapy in non-medicalised ways that are consistent with the basic ethical and theoretical principles of the approach. We propose that the crux of client-centred therapy is the move toward unconditional positive self-regard and thus it is this which should be at the core of research to evaluate client-centred therapy. A number of other measures are also available which promise to be useful in developing theoretically grounded research, although clearly there remains a need for the development of further appropriate measures in the future. We have discussed measures that provide indices of psychological change within the person and we would note that we have therefore not discussed other measures that have been developed, such as the widely validated Barrett-Lennard Relationship Inventory (BLRI); (Barrett-Lennard, 1962) which assesses the quality of the relationship as experienced. Although less useful as an outcome measure of change within the person, the BLRI is a valuable measurement resource that can be used by researchers interested in the differential contribution of the client-centred core relationship conditions of congruence, empathy and unconditional positive regard to therapeutic outcome. Finally, although we call for greater research attention to constructs grounded in and consistent with person-centred theory, until our own research base is more firmly established we do also see a continued role within the current climate of evidence-based practice for research that evaluates client-centred therapy in terms of constructs grounded in psychiatric terminology.

211

REFERENCES

Ackerman, SJ, Benjamin, LS, Beutler, LE, Gelso, C, Goldfried, MR, Hill, C et al. (2001) Empirically supported therapy relationships: conclusions and recommendations of the Division 29 Task Force. *Psychotherapy, 38,* 495–7.

Barrett-Lennard, GT (1962) Dimensions of therapist response as causal factors in therapeutic change. *Psychological Monographs, 76,* 43 (Whole No. 562).

Barrett-Lennard, GT (1986) The Relationship Inventory now: Issues and advances in theory, method, and use. In LS Greenberg and WM Pinsof (eds) *The Psychotherapeutic Process: A research handbook* (pp. 439–76). New York: Guilford Press.

Barrett-Lennard, GT (1998) *Carl Rogers' Helping System: Journey and substance.* London: Sage.

Bentall, RP (2003) *Madness Explained: Psychosis and human nature.* London: Allen Lane.

Betz, NE, Wohlgemuth, E, Serling, D, Harshbarger, J and Klein, K (1995) Evaluation of a measure of self-esteem based on the concept of unconditional self-regard. *Journal of Counseling and Development, 74,* 76–82.

Bohart, AC, O'Hara, M and Leitner, L (1998) Empirically violated treatments: disenfranchisement of humanistic and other psychotherapies. *Psychotherapy Research, 8,* 141–57.

Bozarth, JD (1998) *Person-Centred Therapy: A revolutionary paradigm.* Ross-on-Wye: PCCS Books.

Bozarth, JD (2002) Empirically supported treatment: The epitome of the specificity myth. In J Watson, R Goldman and M Warner (eds) *Client-Centered and Experiential Psychotherapy in the 21st Century: Advances in theory, research, and practice* (pp. 168–81). Ross-on-Wye: PCCS Books.

Bozarth, JD, Zimring, FM and Tausch, R (2002) Client-centered therapy: The evolution of a revolution. In D Cain and J Seeman (eds) *Research in Humanistic Psychology* (pp. 147–88). Washington DC: American Psychological Association.

Brown, KW and Ryan, RM (2003) The benefits of being present: Mindfulness and its role in psychological well-being. *Journal of Personality and Social Psychology, 84,* 822–48.

Brown, KW and Ryan, RM (2004) Fostering healthy self-regulation from within and without: A Self-Determination Theory perspective. In PA Linley and S Joseph (eds) *Positive Psychology in Practice* (pp. 105–24). New York: Wiley.

Butler, JM and Haigh, GV (1954) Changes in the relation between self-concepts and ideal concepts consequent upon client-centred counseling. In CR Rogers and RF Dymond (eds) *Psychotherapy and Personality Change* (pp. 55–75). Chicago: University of Chicago Press.

Carr, AC (1949) An evaluation of psychotherapy cases by means of the Rorschach. *Journal of Consulting Psychology, 13,* 196–205.

Cartwright, D and Mori, C (1988) Scales for assessing aspects of the person. *Person-Centered Review, 3,* 176–94.

Carver, CS (1997) You want to measure coping but your protocol's too long: Consider the brief COPE. *International Journal of Behavioural Medicine, 4,* 92–100.

Cornelius-White, JH (2002) The phoenix of empirically supported therapy relationships: The overlooked person-centered basis. *Psychotherapy: Theory, Research, Practice, Training, 39,* 219–22.

Crocker, J and Wolfe, CT (2001) Contingencies of self-worth. *Psychological Review, 108,* 593–623.

Crocker, J, Luhtanen, RK, Cooper, ML and Bouvrette, A (2003) Contingencies of self-worth in college students: Theory and measurement. *Journal of Personality and Social Psychology, 85,* 894–908.

Elliot, AJ and McGregor, HA (2001) A 2 x 2 achievement goal framework. *Journal of Personality and Social Psychology, 80,* 501–19.

Elliott, R (1996) Are client-centred/experiential therapies effective? A meta-analysis of outcome research. In U Esser, H Pabst, and G-W Speierer (eds) *The Power of the Person-Centered Approach: New challenges-perspectives-answers* (pp. 125–38). Köln: GwG Verlag.

Fox, J, Knapp, R and Michael, W (1968) Assessment of self-actualization of psychiatric patients: Validity of the Personal Orientation Inventory. *Educational and Psychological Measurement, 28,* 565–9.

Friedli, K, King, M, Lloyd, M and Horder, J (1997) Randomised controlled assessment of non-directive psychotherapy versus routine general practitioner care. *The Lancet, 350,* 1662–5.

Gordon, T and Cartwright, D (1954) The effect of psychotherapy upon certain attitudes towards others. In CR Rogers and RF Dymond (eds) *Psychotherapy and Personality Change* (pp. 167–95). Chicago: University of Chicago Press.

Hubble, MA and Miller, SD (2004) The client: Psychotherapy's missing link for promoting a positive psychology. In PA Linley and S Joseph (eds) *Positive Psychology in Practice* (pp. 335–53). Hoboken, NJ: Wiley.

Joseph, S (2003) Person-centred approach to understanding post-traumatic stress. *Person-Centred Practice, 11,* 70–5.

Joseph, S (2004) Client-centred therapy, post-traumatic stress, and post-traumatic growth: Theoretical perspectives and practical implications. *Psychology and Psychotherapy: Theory, Research and Practice, 77,* 101–20.

Joseph, S (2005) Understanding post-traumatic stress from the person-centred perspective. In S Joseph and R Worsley (eds) *Person-Centred Psychopathology: A positive psychology of mental health* (pp. 190–201). Ross-on-Wye: PCCS Books.

Joseph, S and Lewis, CA (1998) The Depression-Happiness Scale: Reliability and validity of a bipolar self-report scale. *Journal of Clinical Psychology, 54,* 537–44.

Joseph, S and Linley, PA (2005) Positive adjustment to threatening events: An organismic valuing theory of growth through adversity. *Review of General Psychology, 9,* 262–80.

Joseph, S, Linley, PA, Andrews, L, Harris, G, Howle, B, Woodward, C, and Shevlin, M (2005) Assessing positive and negative changes in the aftermath of adversity: Psychometric evaluation of the Changes in Outlook Questionnaire. *Psychological Assessment, 17,* 70–80.

Joseph, S, Linley, PA, Harwood, J, Lewis, CA and McCollam, P (2004) Rapid assessment of well-being: The Short Depression–Happiness Scale. *Psychology and Psychotherapy: Theory, Research, and Practice, 77,* 1–14.

Joseph, S, Linley, PA, Shevlin, M, Goodfellow, B, and Butler, L (2006) Assessing positive and negative changes in the aftermath of adversity: A short form of the Changes in Outlook Questionnaire. *Journal of Loss and Trauma, 11,* 85–99.

Joseph, S, Williams, R and Yule, W (1993) Changes in outlook following disaster: The preliminary development of a measure to assess positive and negative responses. *Journal of Traumatic Stress, 6,* 271–9.

Joseph, S and Worsley, R (eds) (2005a) *Person-Centred Psychopathology: A positive psychology of mental health.* Ross-on-Wye: PCCS Books.

Joseph, S and Worsley, R (2005b) A positive psychology of mental health: The person-centred perspective. In S Joseph and R Worsley (eds) *Person-Centred Psychopathology: A positive psychology of mental health* (pp. 348–57). Ross-on-Wye: PCCS Books.

King, M, Sibbald, B, Ward, E, Bower, P, Lloyd, M, Gabbay, M and Byford, S (2000) Randomised controlled trial of non-directive counselling, cognitive behaviour therapy and usual general practitioner care in the management of depression as well as mixed anxiety and depression in primary care. *British Medical Journal, 321*, 1383–8.

King, R (1998) Evidence-based practice: Where is the evidence? The case of cognitive behaviour therapy and depression. *Australian Psychologist, 33*, 83–8.

Kuhn, T (1962/1996) *The Structure of Scientific Revolutions.* Chicago, IL: University of Chicago Press.

Lambert, M (1992) Psychotherapy outcome research. In JC Norcross and MR Goldfried (eds) *Handbook of Psychotherapy Integration* (pp. 94–129). New York: Basic Books.

Lambert, MJ and Barley, DE (2001) Research summary on the therapeutic relationship and psychotherapy outcome. *Psychotherapy, 38*, 357–61.

Lambert, MJ Shapiro, DA and Bergin, AE (1986) The effectiveness of psychotherapy. In SL Garfield and AE Bergin (eds) *Handbook of Psychotherapy and Behavior Change* (pp. 157–212). New York: Wiley.

Lefrancois, R, Leclerc, G, Dube, M, Herbert, R and Gaulin, P (1997) The development and validation of a self-report measure of self-actualisation. *Social Behaviour and Personality, 25*, 353–66.

Luborsky, L, Rosenthal, R, Diguer, L, Andrusyna, TP, Berman, JS, Levitt, JT et al. (2002) The dodo bird verdict is alive and well— mostly. *Clinical Psychology: Science and practice, 9*, 2–12.

Luborsky, L, Singer, B and Luborsky, L (1975) Comparative studies of psychotherapies: Is it true that 'Everyone has won and all must have prizes?' *Archives of General Psychiatry, 32*, 995–1008.

Patterson, CH (1984) Empathy, warmth, and genuineness in psychotherapy: A review of reviews. *Psychotherapy, 26*, 427–35.

Patterson, TG and Joseph, S (2006) Development of a measure of unconditional positive self-regard. *Psychology and Psychotherapy: Theory, research, and practice, 79*, 557–70.

Patterson, TG and Joseph, S (2007) Person-centred personality theory: Support from self-determination theory and positive psychology. *Journal of Humanistic Psychology, 47*, 117–39.

Pfaffenberger, AH (2006) Critical issues in therapy outcome research. *Journal of Humanistic Psychology, 46*, 336–51.

Popper, K (1959/1980) *The Logic of Scientific Discovery.* London: Hutchinson.

Rogers, CR (1951) *Client-Centered Therapy: Its current practice, implications and theory.* Boston: Houghton Mifflin.

Rogers, CR (1957a) The necessary and sufficient conditions of therapeutic personality change. *Journal of Consulting Psychology, 21*, 95–103.

Rogers, CR (1957b) A therapist's view of the good life. *The Humanist, 17*, 291–300.

Rogers, CR (1959) A theory of therapy, personality, and interpersonal relationships as developed in the client-centered framework. In S Koch (ed) *Psychology: A Study of a Science, Vol. 3: Formulations of the person and the social context* (pp. 184–256). New York: McGraw-Hill.

Rogers, CR (1961) *On Becoming a Person.* Boston: Houghton Mifflin.

Rogers, CR (1985) Toward a more human science of the person. *Journal of Humanistic Psychology, 25*, 7–24.

Roth, A and Fonagy, P (1996) *What Works for Whom? A critical review of psychotherapy research.* New York: Guilford.

Sheldon, KM (1995) Creativity and self-determination in personality. *Creativity Research Journal, 8,* 61–72.

Sheldon, KM and Deci, EL (1996) The Self-Determination Scale. Unpublished manuscript, University of Rochester. Rochester, NY.

Sheldon, KM, Ryan, RM and Reis, H (1996) What makes for a good day? Competence and autonomy in the day and in the person. *Personality and Social Psychology Bulletin, 22,* 1270–9.

Shostrom, EL (1966a) A test for the measurement of self-actualization. *Educational and Psychological Measurement, 24,* 207–18.

Shostrom, EL (1966b) *Manual for the POI.* San Diego, CA: Educational and Industrial Testing Service.

Shostrom, EL, and Knapp, RR (1967) The relationship of a measure of self-actualization to a measure of pathology and therapeutic growth. *American Journal of Psychotherapy, 20,* 192–203.

Snyder, WU (1945) An investigation of the nature of non-directive psychotherapy. *Journal of General Psychology, 33,* 193–223.

Sorochan, WD (1976) *Personal Health Appraisal.* New York: Wiley and Sons.

APPENDIX

UNCONDITIONAL POSITIVE SELF-REGARD SCALE (UPSRS)

Section 2: Below is a list of statements dealing with your general feelings about yourself. Please, respond to each statement by circling your answer using the scale 1 = Strongly Disagree to 5 = Strongly Agree.

		Strongly Disagree	Disagree	Unsure	Agree	Strongly Agree
1	I truly like myself.	1	2	3	4	5
2	Whether other people criticise me or praise me makes no real difference to the way I feel about myself.	1	2	3	4	5
3	There are certain things I like about myself and there are other things I don't like.	1	2	3	4	5
4	I feel that I appreciate myself as a person.	1	2	3	4	5
5	Some things I do make me feel good about myself whereas other things I do cause me to be critical of myself.	1	2	3	4	5
6	How I feel towards myself is not dependent on how others feel towards me.	1	2	3	4	5
7	I have a lot of respect for myself.	1	2	3	4	5
8	I feel deep affection for myself.	1	2	3	4	5
9	I treat myself in a warm and friendly way.	1	2	3	4	5
10	I don't think that anything I say or do really changes the way I feel about myself.	1	2	3	4	5
11	I really value myself.	1	2	3	4	5
12	Whether other people are openly appreciative of me or openly critical of me, it does not really change how I feel about myself.	1	2	3	4	5

Scoring Key for the UPSRS*:

Strongly Disagree = 1
Disagree = 2
Unsure = 3
Agree = 4
Strongly Agree = 5
*Items 3 and 5 are reverse scored.

Scores have a possible range of 6 to 30 on each of the two subscales. On the 'Self-Regard' subscale, higher scores indicate greater relative presence of positive self-regard while lower scores indicate greater relative absence of positive self-regard. On the 'Conditionality' subscale, higher scores indicate more *unconditionality* of self-regard, while lower scores indicate more *conditionality* of self-regard.

Subscales:

Items 1 + 4 + 7 + 8 + 9 +11 = Self-Regard Subscale
Items 2 + 3 + 5 + 6 + 10 + 12 = Conditionality Subscale

REFERENCE

Patterson, TG and Joseph, S (2006) Development of a measure of unconditional positive self-regard. *Psychology and Psychotherapy: Theory, research, and practice, 79,* 557–70.

CHAPTER 18

PERSON-CENTRED PRACTICE AND POSITIVE PSYCHOLOGY: CROSSING THE BRIDGES BETWEEN DISCIPLINES

STEPHEN JOSEPH AND RICHARD WORSLEY

As with our previous volume on person-centred psychopathology (Joseph and Worsley, 2005), our aim in developing this book was to bring together experts in the person-centred approach who would write about their work in such a way as to illustrate the meta-theoretical assumption underpinning person-centred practice, i.e., that people are intrinsically motivated toward being fully functioning. In this, we show how this way of thinking could be applied to people suffering from a variety of so-called psychological disorders. From the perspective of person-centred personality theory, there is no absolute distinction between the facilitation of human growth and the relief of distress, for both involve the person becoming more fully and congruently engaged with the processes associated with organismic evaluation. This is what makes the person-centred approach different from other therapeutic approaches and what makes it an exemplar as a positive psychology.

PERSON-CENTRED APPROACH AS POSITIVE PSYCHOLOGY

Historically, the person-centred approach has been seen to belong within the wider humanistic psychology movement, but now we can conceptualise it as part of the wider positive psychology movement as well as an exemplar of what might be described as 'positive therapy' (Joseph and Linley, 2006). As Pete Sanders (Chapter 16) notes, the alignment of person-centred psychology with that of the positive psychology movement provides an opportunity to promote the ideas and values of person-centred psychology within mainstream psychology, and thus to combat the marginalisation of person-centred psychology that has occurred over the last two decades. The term positive psychology is becoming increasingly familiar and refers to the recent movement by psychologists to investigate what makes life worth living, and the development of new ways of working which are focused on the facilitation of well-being (Linley and Joseph, 2004). For too long, positive psychologists claim, the profession of psychology has been focused on pathology, and there is a need, they argue, for equal attention to be paid to what leads to well-being.

This is an admirable goal and as person-centred practitioners we might welcome it because it provides a new opportunity to draw attention to how the person-centred approach has, at its meta-theoretical level, always been equally focused on both the negative and the positive sides of human experience—that is the profound implication of Carl Rogers (1963) adoption of the actualising tendency as '… the one central source of energy in the human organism …' (p. 6).

We are not saying that we should not be concerned with the alleviation of pathology—after all, as counsellors and psychotherapists that is often our role—but what is inherent in the person-centred approach is that, in our endeavour to assist a person who is distressed, our goal is to facilitate their movement toward fully functioning. Thus, whereas it is appropriate for medical-model practitioners to think about therapeutic progress in relation to the amount of psychopathology, for person-centred practitioners it is appropriate to think about therapeutic progress in terms of the congruent engagement with the organismic evaluation process. Medical model practitioners might, for example, use assessment instruments designed to assess the levels of depression, anxiety, and so on—and, as levels of depression and anxiety fall, see that as evidence of effective practice. But for the person-centred practitioner, the effectiveness of what we do should not be judged by these same criteria—we should also be looking to see an increase in functionality: is the person becoming more open to experience, congruent in their relationships, unconditionally self-accepting, and so on? It is these criteria, as Patterson and Joseph (Chapter 17) argue, that person-centred theory sets out as the therapeutic outcome objectives. Rarely, however, is this made explicit in writings on the person-centred approach, which, like other forms of therapy, has tended to discuss therapeutic progress in terms of the alleviation of psychopathology. It was to this theme of positive psychology, as it relates to person-centred practice, that we asked our contributors to write—and it runs as a thread throughout the book.

The themes of positive psychology bring to therapy a particular challenge. While much positive psychology is concerned with what might broadly be termed the promotion of happiness—although the term happiness is not shallow but includes the fullness of existential living—the therapist who deals mainly with those in distress can use positive psychology insights to move beyond the client's distress to a shared appreciation of how clients grow through their experience. Stephen's work on post-traumatic growth is a prime example of this (e.g., Joseph, 2005; Joseph and Linley, 2005). Richard's case study of Emma (Chapter 9) concerns a deeply depressed person's journey towards, not the relief of symptoms, but a creative existential engagement with depression and meaning.

Many of the chapters illustrate the point of how the person-centred approach is a positive psychology but, as editors, we were struck by how carefully we had to encourage our authors to state this theme explicitly. As a result we have begun to wonder whether the person-centred movement has itself become so overawed and besieged by the medical-model ideology that we have, as a profession, lost sight of the alternative paradigmatic nature of our therapeutic approach and have ourselves become overly focused on the alleviation of pathology and less appreciative of the distinct meta-theoretical stance that constitutes the person-centred approach. As practitioners, it may be that living day by day with client distress makes it difficult or even impertinent to look for growth through pain. After all, it is not the therapist who is in immediate pain. Only when we, as person-centred therapists, have a clear conviction and faith in growth through distress will we be able to hear the client's experience of growth.

On reflection, it would not be surprising if we do, all too often, think like medical-model practitioners; after all that is the wider dominant culture that we work within. It will demand of us ways of working that run counter to the principles of person-centred therapy. Employment contexts may demand of us that we offer a service for depression, anxiety, or post-traumatic stress, for example, and as a duty to our employers we are obliged to show that what we do is effective in reducing these psychological complaints. However, with the advent of positive psychology there is the opportunity for the person-centred community to align itself with a broadly similar and powerful new perspective within the dominant culture (see Linley and Joseph, 2004) in which it is also appropriate to look to people's strengths—to see the task of the therapist as one of facilitating movement toward being fully functioning, not just assisting the alleviation of pathology.

It is our hope that this book will serve to tilt the rudder so that, as a profession, we orientate ourselves more explicitly in the direction of what it means to be person-centred, and to embrace the distinct meta-theoretical, positive psychological stance of person-centred theory.

PERSON-CENTRED APPROACH: PSYCHOTHERAPY, COUNSELLING, OR COACHING?

Since we began writing about the links between the person-centred approach and positive psychology, the situation has become even more confused in recent years with the emergence of the professions of coaching and coaching psychology. Coaches and coaching psychologists, like positive psychologists, are concerned with optimal health and the facilitation of strengths, well-being, and happiness.

But coaching has emerged in a culture dominated by the medical model and, as a result, differentiates itself from the world of therapy. It sees itself as promoting growth beyond the mere plateau of functionality to which therapy aspires. Ostensibly, coaches are concerned with people who are already functioning well in the world and want to function more effectively, whereas therapists are concerned with those who are dysfunctional and distressed and want to be cured of their pathology. This split makes sense from the medical-model perspective, but from the person-centred meta-theoretical perspective it does not. Counselling and psychotherapy, as much as coaching, may bring a person towards an actualisation of their potential as human beings at work, in their family or in their inner living.

As these new territorial battles begin to ensue, the person-centred approach, long besieged already by medical-model practitioners for being only useful for the worried well, is now in danger of being besieged by the world of coaching for being a therapy, rather than a way of facilitating optimal functioning. But the person-centred approach is just that: an approach to helping that, in some contexts, could be called psychotherapy, counselling, or coaching. There is a danger that the person-centred profession could be caught between these territorial battles, fuelled by medical-model ideology and squeezed at both ends as if irrelevant. We should not be distracted by the differences in terminology. What the person-centred approach offers is a unified way of working across the spectrum of human experience (see Joseph, 2006).What is distinctive about the person-centred approach is its meta-theoretical stance.

PERSON-CENTRED RESEARCH

Thus, the person-centred community needs to engage with the wider research culture. Certainly, an issue in the past has been the reluctance to engage with medical-model-based research in order to investigate the effectiveness of person-centred therapy for the range of so called psychiatric disorders—as to do so contravenes the theoretical premise of the person-centred approach. But where is the *alternative* research, consistent with the person-centred approach, showing that it *does* lead to a movement toward being fully functioning? A wealth of psychological tests and measures have been developed within the history of humanistic psychology (and more recently positive psychology) to allow for the investigation of subjective and psychological well-being. We need to begin to embrace the culture of evidence-based practice, recognising that this does not imply that we also embrace medical model ideology.

The person-centred approach has often been criticised for its lack of research by those working in the medical model perspective who fail to appreciate the phenomenological nature of the approach and the clinical validity of qualitative research. Certainly, in addressing the need for research, we do need to ensure that we continue to make the case for phenomenology and qualitative research, but we do also need to engage with the wider research community using quantitative psychological methods. But it is incorrect to say that the research evidence is non-existent. There is a rich heritage of research in the person-centred tradition (see Barrett-Lennard, 1998); a wealth of psychotherapy research documenting the importance of the relationship (Wampold, 2001); randomised controlled trials supportive of person-centred therapy (King et al., 2000); and a convergence of positive psychological research and theory supportive of person-centred approach (Patterson and Joseph, 2007).

Because of the holistic and phenomenological nature of person-centred therapy, outcome research, done as a mere measure of client change in relation to outcomes defined through a medical model ideology, is not enough. Those who regulate or fund therapy need to understand exactly what the power of the approach is in clients with widely varying degrees of distress—not to mention the genius of the approach to foster positive existential growth which transcends mere symptom alleviation. As Patterson and Joseph (Chapter 17) argue, there is a need for empirical research that adopts outcome measures consistent with person-centred theory, such as the assessment of unconditional positive self-regard. But in addition, case studies have a particular and important part to play. They exemplify the varied workings of mature practitioners. They illustrate the huge resource for change in the approach. They demonstrate that person-centred therapy is neither shallow work with the worried well, nor long-drawn-out work suitable only for private practice. But, above all, they demonstrate that clients have the innate ability to find real growth beyond the relief of symptoms.

Those who know the work of Margaret Warner will be aware that the case of Luke has preoccupied her over many years. She has been admirably committed to reflecting consistently—even tenaciously—upon one case, so that she and we, may learn in depth. (Chapter 13).

Human growth happens in context. It is not a vague ideal, nor is it to be seen as trapped within the perspective of relentless individualism. In short, the person-centred approach, and its shared vision with positive psychology, is of socio-political significance. Within this volume, this is amply illustrated by the argument put forward by Pete Sanders that therapy is rooted in community action (Chapter 16) and by Tracey Sanders and June O'Brien, that the approach is a particular resource for those who are socially disadvantaged (Chapter 5). When the person-centred approach maintains its alertness to its own meta-theory and its rootedness in relationship and community, it becomes politically and spiritually alive, militant and active.

TRAINING AND PRACTICE

Aside from the above theoretical issues, this book provides a much needed look at what person-centred practitioners do. In our experience, beginning therapists to the approach do find it difficult to get a sense of what person-centred therapy looks like in practice. What does the person-centred therapist actually do? It is not much use to the new practitioner to explain that the therapist endeavours to be empathic, congruent and unconditionally accepting. Other technique-based approaches to therapy have a clear 'sales' advantage and can often more readily appeal to the novice therapist looking for a quick answer to the question of 'what do I do?' As Alex Payne has made clear (Chapter 2), the issue of 'what I do' is made so much more pertinent for those training in, for example, clinical psychology. Clinical psychology adopts a medical-model approach, insofar as trainees are expected to know different therapeutic techniques appropriate to the treatment of different psychological problems. Thus, the person-centred approach can often seem irrelevant to those training in clinical psychology because it doesn't address this 'need to know what to do' in different contexts. It is for this need that we hope the present volume will be useful.

However, even in counsellor training (which is not necessarily rooted at all in the medical model, save for the cultural presuppositions of the whole of the Western world) it is important for beginning counsellors to have a view *over the shoulder*, as it were, of mature practitioners. Person-centred training is certainly not about learning techniques. It is a growth in faith in relating. The case studies in this book will nurture this faith in trainees. Beyond person-centred training courses, we hope that at a practical level other approaches will come to experience and understand with clarity the philosophy and practice of the approach—for person-centred therapy is often misunderstood, misrepresented, stereotyped and sold short.

In looking across the chapters at what therapists do, we are struck by the diversity of practice that co-exists under the umbrella of the person-centred. The truth is simply that the attitudinal conditions of empathy, congruence, and unconditional positive regard cannot be manualised and that every therapist will express their attitudes in their own idiosyncratic way. If we accept that it is the human relationship that is central to healing in psychotherapy then it is inevitable that therapy is sometimes messy, sometimes clumsy, and that this is simply the nature of it. We take heart in hearing the accounts provided in this volume, their stories of when things went wrong, their reflections on their practice, and hope that others too will find these cases similarly encouraging. Above all, we (and we suspect all other authors in this volume) practise person-centred therapy out of a depth of love for both our clients and the process of growth.

REFERENCES

Barrett-Lennard, GT (1998) *Carl Rogers' Helping System: Journey and substance*. London: Sage.

Joseph, S (2005) Understanding post-traumatic stress from the person-centred perspective. In S Joseph and R Worsley (eds) *Person-Centred Psychopathology* (pp. 190–201). Ross-on-Wye: PCCS Books.

Joseph, S (2006) Person-centred coaching psychology: A meta-theoretical perspective. *International Coaching Psychology Review, 1*, 47–54.

Joseph, S and Linley, PA (2005) Positive adjustment to threatening events: An organismic valuing theory of growth through adversity. *Review of General Psychology, 9*, 262–80.

Joseph, S and Linley, PA (2006) *Positive Therapy: A meta-theory for positive psychological practice*. London: Routledge.

Joseph, S and Worsley R (eds) (2005) *Person-Centred Psychopathology: A positive psychology of mental health*. Ross-on-Wye: PCCS Books.

King, M, Sibbald, B, Ward, E, Bower, P, Lloyd, M, Gabbay, M and Byford, S (2000) Randomised, controlled trial of non-directive counselling, cognitive behaviour therapy and usual general practitioner care in the management of depression, as well as mixed anxiety and depression in primary care. *British Medical Journal, 321*, 1383–8.

Linley, PA and Joseph, S (eds) (2004) *Positive Psychology in Practice*. Hoboken, NJ: John Wiley and Sons, Inc.

Patterson, T and Joseph, S (2007) Person-centered personality theory: Support from self-determination theory and positive psychology. *Journal of Humanistic Psychology, 47*, 117–39.

Rogers, CR (1963) The actualizing tendency in relation to 'motives' and to consciousness. In M. Jones (ed) *Nebraska Symposium on Motivation, Vol. 11* (pp. 1–24). Lincoln: University of Nebraska Press.

Wampold, BE (2001) *The Great Psychotherapy Debate: Models, methods, and findings*. Mahwah, NJ: Lawrence Erlbaum.

CONTRIBUTORS

EDITORS

Stephen Joseph, PhD, is Professor of Psychology, Health & Social Care at the University of Nottingham, where he is co-director of the Centre for Trauma, Resilience and Growth, and an Honorary Consultant Psychologist in Psychotherapy in Nottinghamshire Healthcare NHS Trust. Stephen is a senior practitioner member of the British Psychological Society's Register of Psychologists who specialise in Psychotherapy. Stephen's research interests are in the study of traumatic stress, resilience, and growth following adversity, and in positive psychological applications to therapy.

Richard Worsley is a person-centred counsellor, trainer and supervisor with particular interests in process work and the philosophy and spirituality of counselling, as well as in group work. He works as a staff and student counsellor at the University of Warwick. He has worked for many years as an Anglican priest, with a research interest in philosophical theology. He has written on process work, on integration, on spirituality and on philosophy and counselling, as well as on the theological problem of evil.

CONTRIBUTORS

Jerold Bozarth, PhD, learned client-centered therapy from working with chronic psychotic, hospitalized clients. He has published over 300 articles and book chapters and three books, and has consulted with person-centered training programs in Austria, Brazil, Czech Republic, England, Portugal and Slovakia. He is Professor Emeritus of the University of Georgia and a member of the Golden Pantry Coffee Club.

Matthew Campling is a BACP accredited therapist. He has been an advice writer (agony uncle) to various publications and a regular guest expert on ITV's 'Trisha' show. He also works in management development and support and facilitates groups on his eating disorder recovery approach. Contact at <www. eatingdisorderself-cure.com>.

Elaine Catterall is an accredited person-centred counsellor and works independently for several agencies; counselling children, adolescents and adults. She describes her work as being firmly boundaried by person-centred theory but remains open to other theories if they expand her self-awareness.

Ann Glauser received her PhD from the University of Georgia in Counseling and Human Development Services. She studied with Jerold Bozarth and worked with him on person-centered projects including the initiation of the person-centered workshop in Warm Springs, Georgia. Ann is an associate professor and counselor at the University of Georgia where she teaches and counsels with students experiencing academic difficulties. She has incorporated the principles of the person-centered approach across the curriculum of courses that she has developed and taught for the past twenty years. Her current research interests relate to extra-therapeutic variables (internal and external client resources) in the counseling process and the development of psycho-educational approaches to teaching.

Jan Hawkins is a person-centred practitioner, supervisor and freelance trainer. In 1994 Jan created and co-facilitated a Diploma course in Counselling Survivors of Childhood Abuse, the first initiative of its kind in Europe. For the past five years, through FDP, Jan has continued to run Accredited (Middlesex University) post-counselling training Diploma courses with a conviction that experiential learning is an imperative for developing empathy as well as skills.

Barbara Krietemeyer works in Germany as a psychologist and psychotherapist. She practises the person-centred approach in a facility for people with mental disabilities and persons with brain injuries.

Brian E. Levitt, PsyD, CPsych, trained for several years at the Chicago Counseling and Psychotherapy Center and the Pre-Therapy Institute. He practises in Ontario, Canada as a Rehabilitation and Clinical Psychologist. Brian is the editor of *Embracing Non-Directivity* (PCCS books).

Thomas Patterson is a Clinical Psychologist at Coventry and Warwickshire Partnership Trust, working across Adult and Older People's specialties. His research interests include the non-medicalised evaluation of therapeutic outcome, and areas of convergence between mainstream academic psychology and person-centred theory.

Alex Payne is a Clinical Psychologist at Reaside Clinic, the West Midlands (UK) Men's Forensic Psychiatry Service. She works with men who experience co-morbid difficulties with mental health problems and violent behaviour. She has a keen interest in Pre-Therapy.

Gillian Proctor, DClinPsych, is a Clinical Psychologist with Bradford and Airedale Teaching PCT and an honorary research fellow at the Centre for Citizenship and Community Mental health at the University of Bradford. Publications include: author of *The Dynamics of Therapy in Counselling and Psychotherapy* (2002: PCCS Books); co-editor of *Encountering Feminism* (2004: PCCS Books) and *Politicizing the Person-Centred Approach* (2006: PCCS books). She is currently enjoying exploring the nature of dog-centred relationships with her nearly two-year-old puppy!

Garry Prouty was trained in Person-Centered / Experiential Psychotherapy by Eugene Gendlin of the University of Chicago. He developed his own therapeutic approach at clinics and hospitals dealing with psychotic and retarded clients. Dr Prouty was a Fellow of the Chicago Counseling, Psychotherapy and Research Center. He is the founder of the Pre-Therapy International Network, a European organization working with psychotic persons. He has published numerous books and articles. His most important publication is a 50-year research survey of humanistic psychotherapy with schizophrenics.

Ann Regan works in the community with people with learning difficulties. She is also a complementary therapist specialising in reiki. She has three children and a granddaughter.

Pete Sanders retired from practice in 2003 after more than 25 years as a counsellor, trainer and supervisor. He continues to have an active interest in the politics of therapy, the development of the theory and practice of client-/person-centered therapy, and mental health issues internationally, nationally and where he lives in Herefordshire, UK.

Tracey Sanders is currently the Course Director for the Postgraduate Diploma in Counselling at the University of Strathclyde. Her interests include the impact of social inequality, suicide, spirituality—and raising guide dog puppies.

Martin van Kalmthout, PhD, is a person-centred psychotherapist in private practice. He has published widely about psychotherapy in general and person-centred therapy in particular. He is especially interested in the contribution of the person-centred approach to the meaning of life.

Dion Van Werde is a clinical psychologist and person-centred psychotherapist. He coordinates the Pre-Therapy International Network and translated Prouty's Pre-Therapy into a multidisciplinary ward philosophy and practice in residential care in Ghent, Belgium.

Margaret Warner, PhD, is a Professor and a co-chair of the Minor and Certificate programs in Client-Centered and Experiential Psychotherapies at the Illinois School of Professional Psychology at Argosy University, Chicago. She trained in client-centered therapy at the Chicago Counseling Center, an offshoot of the original Counseling Center founded by Carl Rogers.

INDEX